# Water and Health in an Overcrowded World

## Introducing Health Sciences: A Case Study Approach

Series editor: Basiro Davey

Seven case studies on major topics in global public health are the subject of this multidisciplinary series of books, each with its own animations, videos and learning activities on DVD. They focus on: access to clean water in an overcrowded and polluted world; the integration of psychological and biological approaches to pain; alcohol consumption and its effects on the body; the science, risks and benefits of mammography screening for early breast cancer; chronic lung disease due to smoke pollution – a forgotten cause of millions of deaths worldwide; traffic-related injuries, tissue repair and recovery; and the causes and consequences of visual impairment in developed and developing countries. Each topic integrates biology, chemistry, physics and psychology with health statistics and social studies to illuminate the causes of disease and disability, their impacts on individuals and societies and the science underlying common treatments. These case studies will be of value to anyone who is, or wants to be, working in a health-related occupation where scientific knowledge could enhance your prospects. If you have a wide-ranging interest in human sciences and want to learn more about global health issues and statistics, how the body works and the scientific rationale for screening procedures and treatments, this series is for you.

### Titles in this series

*Water and Health in an Overcrowded World*, edited by Tim Halliday and Basiro Davey

*Pain*, edited by Frederick Toates

*Alcohol and Human Health*, edited by Lesley Smart

*Screening for Breast Cancer*, edited by Elizabeth Parvin

*Chronic Obstructive Pulmonary Disease: A Forgotten Killer*, edited by Carol Midgley

*Trauma, Repair and Recovery*, edited by James Phillips

*Visual Impairment: A Global View*, edited by Heather McLannahan

# Water and Health in an Overcrowded World

Edited by Tim Halliday and Basiro Davey

 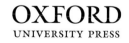

The Open University

OXFORD
UNIVERSITY PRESS

Published by Oxford University Press, Great Clarendon Street, Oxford OX2 6DP
in association with The Open University, Walton Hall, Milton Keynes MK7 6AA.

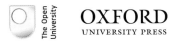

**OXFORD**
UNIVERSITY PRESS

Oxford University Press is a department of the University of Oxford. It furthers the University's
objective of excellence in research, scholarship, and education by publishing worldwide in

Oxford New York
Auckland Cape Town Dar es Salaam Hong Kong Karachi Kuala Lumpur Madrid Melbourne
Mexico City Nairobi New Delhi Shanghai Taipei Toronto

with offices in
Argentina Austria Brazil Chile Czech Republic France Greece Guatemala Hungary
Italy Japan Poland Portugal Singapore South Korea Switzerland
Thailand Turkey Ukraine Vietnam

Oxford is a registered trade mark of Oxford University Press in the UK and in certain
other countries.

Published in the United States by Oxford University Press Inc., New York

First published 2007. Reprinted 2010

Copyright © 2007 The Open University

Edited, and designed by The Open University.

Typeset by SR Nova Pvt. Ltd, Bangalore India.

Printed and bound in the United Kingdom by Latimer Trend & Company Ltd, Plymouth.

This book forms part of the Open University course SDK125 *Introducing Health Sciences: A Case
Study Approach*. Details of this and other Open University courses can be obtained from the Student
Registration and Enquiry Service, The Open University, PO Box 197, Milton Keynes MK7 6BJ,
United Kingdom:
tel. +44 (0)870 333 4340, email general-enquiries@open.ac.uk.

http://www.open.ac.uk

British Library Cataloguing in Publication Data available on request

Library of Congress Cataloging in Publication Data available on request

ISBN 9780 1992 3730 2

10 9 8 7 6 5 4 3 2 1

1.2

The paper used in this
publication contains pulp
sourced from forests
independently certified to the
Forest Stewardship Council
(FSC) principles and criteria.
Chain of custody certification
allows the pulp from these
forests to be tracked to the end
use (see www.fsc.org).

# ABOUT THIS BOOK

This book and the accompanying material on DVD present the first case study in a series of seven, under the collective title *Introducing Health Sciences: A Case Study Approach*. Together they form an Open University (OU) course for students beginning the first year of an undergraduate programme in Health Sciences. Each case study has also been designed to 'stand alone' for readers studying it in isolation from the rest of the course, either as part of an educational programme at another institution, or for general interest and self-directed study.

*Water and Health in an Overcrowded World* is a multidisciplinary introduction to a topic of global importance for public health. This case study is for anyone seeking a scientific understanding of human health and the impact on health of the environments in which people live, particularly their access to clean, safe drinking water. In such a wide-ranging subject area, we have had to be selective, but we have included aspects of the biology, chemistry, psychology and epidemiology of the topic, as indicated in the contents list at the start of the book. No previous experience of studying science has been assumed and new concepts and specialist terminology are explained with examples and illustrations. There is some mathematical content; the emphasis is mainly on interpreting data in tables and graphs, but the text also introduces you step-by-step to some ways of performing calculations that are commonly used in science.

To help you plan your study of this material, we have included a number of 'icons' in the margin to indicate different types of activity which have been included to help you develop and practise particular skills. This icon indicates when to undertake an activity on the accompanying DVD. You will need to 'run' the DVD programs on your computer because they are *interactive,* and this function doesn't operate on a domestic DVD-player. The DVD presents three guided activities: the first explains how bacteria evolve resistance to common antibiotics; the second introduces the chemistry of the water molecule and some of the contaminants of drinking water, and the third examines chemical compounds released into the environment that affect health because they resemble the female hormone, oestrogen.

Activities involving pencil-and-paper exercises are indicated by this icon , and if you need a calculator you will see . Some additional activities for Open University students only are described in a *Companion* text, which is not available outside the OU course. These are indicated by this icon in the margin. Some activities involve using the internet and are marked by this icon . References to activities for OU students are given in the margins of the book and should not interrupt your concentration if you are not studying it as part of an OU course.

At various points in the book, you will find 'boxed' material of two types: Explanation Boxes and Enrichment Boxes. The Explanation Boxes contain basic concepts explained in the kind of detail that someone who is completely new to the health sciences is likely to want. The Enrichment Boxes contain extension material, included for added interest, particularly if you already have some knowledge of basic science. If you are studying this book as part of an

OU course, you should note that the Explanation Boxes contain material that is *essential* to your learning and which therefore may be *assessed*. However, the content of the Enrichment Boxes will *not* be tested in the course assessments.

The authors' intention is to bring you into the subject, develop confidence through activities and guidance, and provide a stepping stone into further study. The most important terms appear in **bold** font in the text at the point where they are first defined, and these terms are also in bold in the index at the end of the book. Understanding of the meaning and uses of the bold terms is essential (i.e. assessable) if you are an OU student.

Active engagement with the material throughout this book is encouraged by numerous 'in text' questions, indicated by a diamond symbol (◆), followed immediately by our suggested answers. It is good practice always to cover the answer and attempt your own response to the question before reading ours. At the end of each chapter, there is a summary of the key points and a list of the main learning outcomes, followed by self-assessment questions to enable you to test your own learning. The answers to these questions are at the back of the book. The great majority of the learning outcomes should be achievable by anyone who has studied this book and its DVD material; one or two learning outcomes for some chapters are only achievable by OU students who have completed the *Companion* activities, and these are clearly identified.

### Internet database (ROUTES)

A large amount of valuable information is available via the internet. To help OU students and other readers of books in this series to access good quality sites without having to search for hours, the OU has developed a collection of internet resources on a searchable database called ROUTES. All websites included in the database are selected by academic staff or subject-specialist librarians. The content of each website is evaluated to ensure that it is accurate, well presented and regularly updated. A description is included for each of the resources.

The website address for ROUTES is: http://routes.open.ac.uk/

Entering the Open University course code 'SDK125' in the search box will retrieve all the resources that have been recommended for this book. Alternatively if you want to search for any resources on a particular subject, type in the words which best describe the subject you are interested in (for example, 'water supply'), or browse the alphabetical list of subjects.

## Authors' acknowledgements

As ever in The Open University, this book and DVD combine the efforts of many people with specialist skills and knowledge in different disciplines. The principal authors were (text) Tim Halliday (biology) and Basiro Davey (public health), and (DVD) Hilary MacQueen (biology) and David Roberts (chemistry). Our contributions have been shaped and immeasurably enriched by the OU course team who helped us to plan the content and made numerous comments and suggestions for improvements as the material progressed through several drafts. It would be impossible to thank everyone personally, but we would like to acknowledge the help and support of academic colleagues who have contributed to this book (in alphabetical order of discipline): Nicolette Habgood, Heather McLannahan, Carol Midgley and James Phillips (biology), Lesley Smart (chemistry), Jeanne Katz (health & social care), Elizabeth Parvin (physics) and Frederick Toates (psychology).

The media developers who contributed directly to the production of the DVD programs were Greg Black, Eleanor Crabb and Brian Richardson. Audiovisual material for Open University students was developed by Owen Horn and Jo Mack (Sound and Vision) and by Basiro Davey, Tim Halliday and Carol Midgley. Activities to support Open University students in developing ICT and information literacy skills were devised by Dave Horan (iSkills Project), Clari Hunt (OU Library), Jamie Daniels (web developer) and Basiro Davey.

We are very grateful to our External Assessor, Professor Susan Standring, Head of Department of Anatomy and Human Sciences, Kings College London, whose detailed comments have contributed to the structure and content of the book and kept the needs of our intended readership to the fore.

Special thanks are due to all those involved in the OU production process, chief among them Joy Wilson and Dawn Partner, our wonderful Course Manager and Course Team Assistant, whose commitment, efficiency and unflagging good humour were at the heart of the endeavour. We also warmly acknowledge the contributions of our editor, Bina Sharma, whose skill has improved every aspect of this book; Steve Best, our graphic artist, who developed and drew all the diagrams; Sarah Hofton, our graphic designer, who devised the page designs and layouts; and Martin Keeling, who carried out picture research and rights clearance. The media project managers were Judith Pickering and James Davies.

For the copublication process, we would especially like to thank Jonathan Crowe of Oxford University Press and, from within The Open University, Christianne Bailey (Media Developer, Copublishing). As is the custom, any small errors or shortcomings that have slipped in (despite our collective best efforts) remain the responsibility of the authors. We would be pleased to receive feedback on the book (favourable or otherwise). Please write to the address below.

Dr Basiro Davey, SDK125 Course Team Chair

Department of Biological Sciences
The Open University
Walton Hall
Milton Keynes
MK7 6AA
United Kingdom

*Environmental statement*

Paper and board used in this publication is FSC certified.

Forestry Stewardship Council (FSC) is an independent certification, which certifies that the virgin pulp used to make the paper/board comes from traceable and sustainable sources from well-managed forests.

# CONTENTS

The DVD activities associated with this book were written, designed and developed by Steve Best, Greg Black, Eleanor Crabb, Basiro Davey, Hilary MacQueen, Brian Richardson, David Roberts and Bina Sharma.

# CHAPTER 1

# LIVING IN THE HUMAN ZOO

*The modern human animal is no longer living in conditions natural for his species. Trapped, not by a zoo collector, but by his own brainy brilliance, he has set himself up in a huge, restless menagerie where he is in constant danger of cracking under the strain.*

(Desmond Morris, *The Human Zoo*, 1969)

## 1.1    Introduction

Health, illness, disability and death are matters of immense concern to every person, both as individuals and as members of families and societies. People rely on each other and on the provision of local resources to improve health, prevent disease and injury, and to treat sickness. Population health is also a major preoccupation of governments worldwide, who know that a nation's wealth depends largely on the health of its workforce. On a global scale, international agencies such as the United Nations (UN) and the World Health Organization (WHO) seek to document and redress inequalities in health between countries and between richer and poorer people within societies.

This book takes a global perspective and considers aspects of human health that affect humanity as a whole. The emphasis, as the book's title indicates, is on 'water and health in an overcrowded world'. The first chapter sets contemporary patterns of mortality and illness in a historical context, seeking the origins of the present human condition in the biological and cultural evolution of the human species. It considers the costs and benefits of living in a rapidly urbanising environment, including the emergence of antibiotic-resistant bacteria. Chapter 2 introduces some striking health statistics and uses examples from different regions and countries to illustrate the inequalities in health referred to above. Finally, Chapter 3 describes some of the major health issues associated with lack of access to clean water. The water molecule is explored as a chemical entity and as a vital natural resource, which is too often contaminated with pollutants from human settlements and industrial processes. Interactive multimedia activities illustrate some of these aspects and can be found on the DVD associated with this book.

## 1.2    The modern human environment

### 1.2.1 The transition to agriculture

At some time during 2006 or 2007 the expanding human population of the Earth reached a significant point; for the first time in human history, more people were living in cities and other urban environments than in the countryside. This marks a new stage of a trend in human evolution which began about 12 000 years ago, when ancestral humans began to switch from a nomadic lifestyle and live in permanent settlements. Prior to this point, all humans had lived as hunter-gatherers in groups of about 25 individuals (Lewin, 1999), roaming over large areas of land in search of plant and animal food, as some isolated peoples still do today (Figure 1.1).

The features of human *anatomy* and *physiology* (i.e. the *structures* of the human body and the ways in which they *function*) that exist today are very like those of our hunter-gatherer ancestors, but today's environment is very different to the conditions in which our bodies evolved. In our ancestral environment, food was scarce and widely distributed. Humans were potential prey to predators such as lions, and shelter from extremes of weather would have been limited and temporary. The change to living in settled communities and permanent dwellings brought many benefits; it enabled humans to build fences to keep out predators and to adopt **agriculture**. This was the so-called 'first agricultural revolution' when the growing of crops in prepared land began. About 10 000 years ago, settlers also began to domesticate animals to provide more reliable sources of food (Figure 1.2). This change occurred in several places and at different times (Figure 1.3) and is still occurring in some parts of the world (Figure 1.4, overleaf).

The transition from a nomadic lifestyle into rural settlements and the development of towns and cities is an inexorable 'one-way' process all over the world. But the changed lifestyle has come at a price. Section 1.3 looks briefly at human anatomy and examines the idea that some of the health problems that afflict people today result from the fact that we live in environments that are very different from those in which we evolved. Section 1.4 summarises the costs and benefits of urban living. Next we turn to the process of urbanisation itself.

We will say more about the processes of evolutionary change later in the chapter.

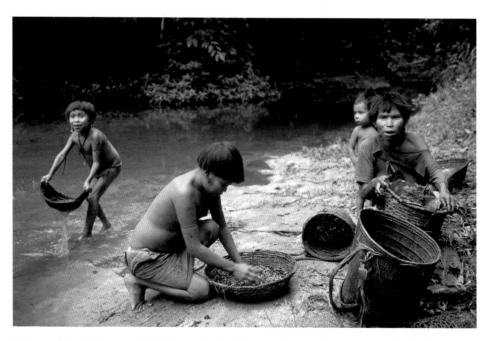

**Figure 1.1**   Yanomani Indians of the Venezuelan and Brazilian rainforests live by fishing, hunting and gathering plants, berries and nuts. This family are catching shellfish from the Orinoco river. (Photo: Mark Edwards/Still Pictures)

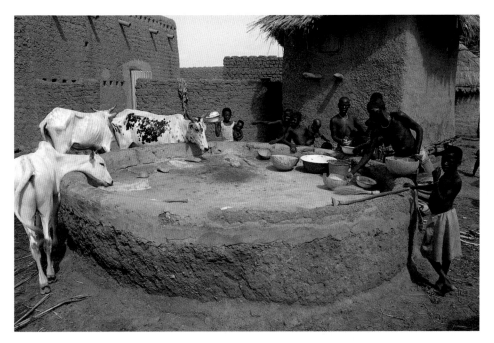

**Figure 1.2** Settlements such as this in the West African state of Burkina Faso provide protection for people and their animals, but their close proximity carries its own health risks. (Photo: Jeremy Hartley/Panos Pictures)

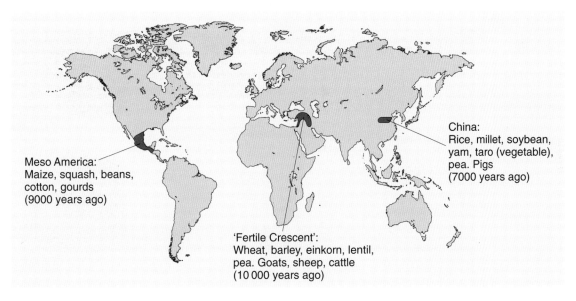

Meso America:
Maize, squash, beans, cotton, gourds
(9000 years ago)

'Fertile Crescent':
Wheat, barley, einkorn, lentil, pea. Goats, sheep, cattle
(10 000 years ago)

China:
Rice, millet, soybean, yam, taro (vegetable), pea. Pigs
(7000 years ago)

**Figure 1.3** Major centres of agricultural innovation. The domestication of animals and plants occurred at different times and in different places. From three major centres, a settled lifestyle based on agriculture spread around the world. The region labelled Meso America refers to an area in which a number of ancient civilisations (including the Aztec and Maya peoples) converged from around 9000 years ago. (Source: Lewin, 1999, p. 216)

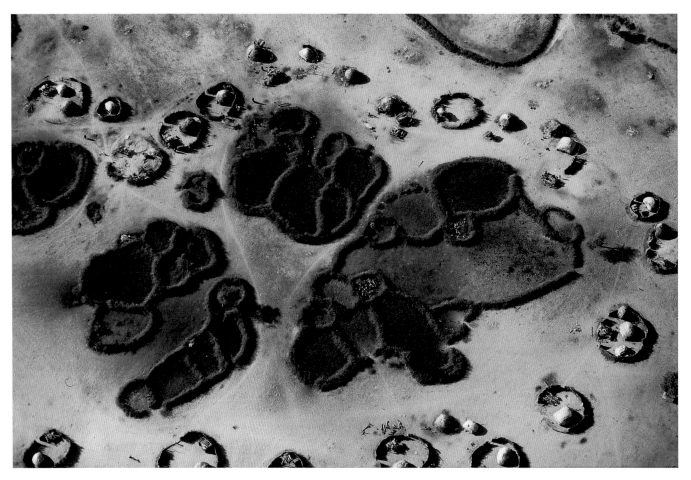

**Figure 1.4** Peul village near Timbuktu, Mali, is a recent example of the transition from a nomadic to a settled lifestyle, following droughts in Mali in 1973–1975 and 1983–1985. The dark brown areas bordered by hedges contain livestock or crops. The darkest soil is due to animal faeces, which fertilise the soil for the growing of crops. (Photo: Arthus-Bertrand)

### 1.2.2 Urbanisation

The urban environment is the furthest removed from that of our ancestral past, and the quotation at the beginning of this chapter from Desmond Morris's influential book claims that it is akin to living in a human zoo (Figure 1.5). When you visit a zoo, you see animals living in an environment that is very different from the natural habitat in which they evolved. They live in a very limited space, protected from natural enemies; they don't have to forage or hunt for their food, and many are forced to live in social groups that are very different from those in which they live in nature. Most animals in zoos live longer than their wild counterparts; elephants are a rare exception. Most, however, require frequent attention from keepers and vets and they may show severe behavioural disorders. Many animals, for example big cats and polar bears, show prolonged repetitive behaviour, called *stereotypy*, in which they pace up and down along a rigidly fixed path.

The life expectancy or longevity (lon-jev-itee) of humans has increased by 30 to 40 years since the great majority gave up a nomadic existence. In this respect, agriculture and **urbanisation** (the movement of people into towns and cities built on land that was once fields, forests or wilderness) has improved the quality of human life, just as living in a zoo enables many animals to live longer. It does not follow, however, that modern humans enjoy better health than our hunter-gathering ancestors, whether they live in managed agricultural landscapes (Figure 1.6) or in towns and cities.

### 1.2.3 The population explosion

At the time of the first agricultural revolution (from about 10 000 years ago), the global human population began to increase, a process that has continued ever since and which has rapidly gathered pace in the last 200 years. Population growth may have hastened the transition from hunter-gathering by increasing the competition for food; perhaps nomadic livelihoods were no longer 'cost-effective' as food-for-free became scarce. Note that drought, which would have reduced natural food supplies, seems to have triggered the Peul people to withdraw into settlements (Figure 1.4).

There is no doubt that the agricultural way of life also led to such an improvement in the food supply that the population was able to increase, but there are alternative views on how this was brought about. The most obvious explanation is that it led to an increase in the *fertility rate* (i.e. the number of babies born per 1000 women of childbearing age).

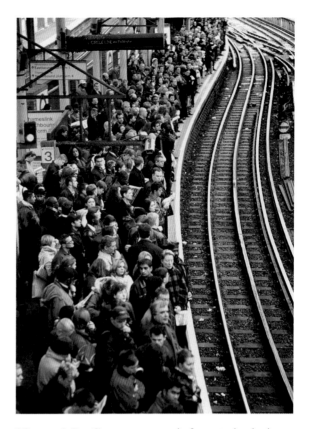

**Figure 1.5** Commuters wait for a train during the morning rush hour, Farringdon Station, England. Humans now live in an environment that is very different from the habitat in which they evolved. (Photo: Phillip Wolmuth/Panos Pictures)

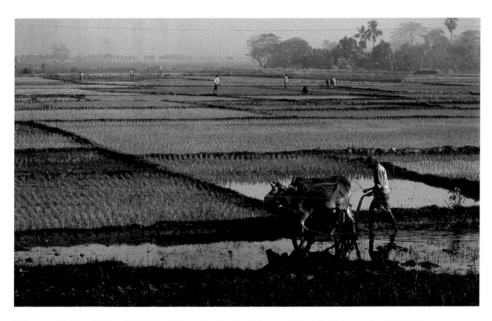

**Figure 1.6** Rice fields in Bangladesh. (Photo: Shoeb Faruquie/DRIK)

◆ Can you suggest some reasons why? (There is more than one.)

◆ A more secure and plentiful food supply would have increased the health of women and improved their likelihood of giving birth to more babies with better survival chances. You may also know that the onset of menstrual periods is delayed in underweight girls, so better nutrition would have made them fertile at an earlier age.

There are two other reasons that are trickier to discern. The availability of cereals stored through the winter enabled the earlier weaning of babies; breast feeding reduces fertility, so weaning babies at an earlier age increases the chance of becoming pregnant again sooner. Also stored food represents a form of wealth and evidence of 'marriageability'; it is likely that in times of plenty, the rate of marriage (or its equivalent) went up and the age at which people married went down, so they had more children during their lifetime. A larger number of surviving children in one generation means more adults to produce an even larger number in the next.

However, a rising birth rate does not equate with a healthier population overall. The fossil remains of early agricultural people indicate that they were, on average, *shorter* by about 10 centimetres (cm) and about 7 kilograms (kg) *lighter* than their hunter-gatherer ancestors. Remains of their bones show that they were susceptible to skeletal diseases, such as rickets ('bowed' long bones in the legs) and osteoporosis (a condition that makes bones brittle), which in younger people are signs of malnutrition (Dunbar, 1991). Agriculture is not a wholly reliable way of producing food, being subject to the vagaries of the climate; drought and flooding lead to crop failure and the death of livestock.

◆ What other adverse effects on health would have resulted from living in communities such as those pictured in Figures 1.2 and 1.4?

◆ The close proximity between humans and their domesticated animals, and the piling up of excrement and other waste in settled areas, led to a huge rise in infectious disease.

Thus, the agricultural revolution appears to have led to a deterioration in human health, paradoxically at the same time as an increased birth rate. The global population grew because the increase in births outnumbered the increase in deaths. In the 19th and early 20th centuries, gradual improvements in human habitation, water supply, sanitation and health care increased the survival of people in many parts of the world, and the population 'explosion' took off (Figure 1.7).

One consequence of the diversity in modern human environments (some of which are illustrated in the photographs in this chapter) is that people living different lives face different health problems, and there are wide variations in their risk of developing the diseases and disabilities that are present in all populations (as Chapter 2 describes). But first, consider the impact of agriculture and urbanisation on the global environment.

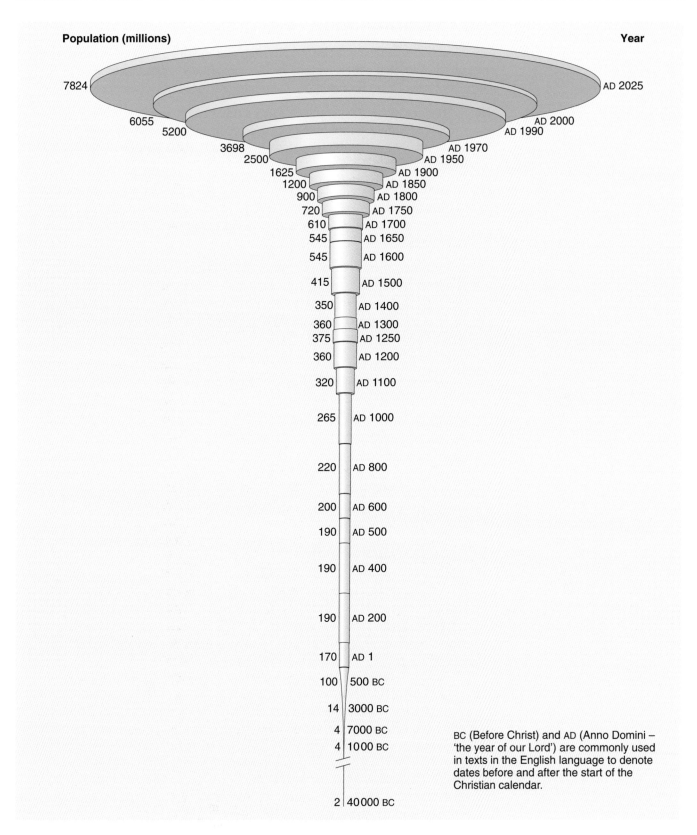

**Population (millions)**  **Year**

7824 — AD 2025
6055 — AD 2000
5200 — AD 1990
3698 — AD 1970
2500 — AD 1950
1625 — AD 1900
1200 — AD 1850
900 — AD 1800
720 — AD 1750
610 — AD 1700
545 — AD 1650
545 — AD 1600
415 — AD 1500
350 — AD 1400
360 — AD 1300
375 — AD 1250
360 — AD 1200
320 — AD 1100
265 — AD 1000
220 — AD 800
200 — AD 600
190 — AD 500
190 — AD 400
190 — AD 200
170 — AD 1
100 — 500 BC
14 — 3000 BC
4 — 7000 BC
4 — 1000 BC
2 — 40 000 BC

BC (Before Christ) and AD (Anno Domini – 'the year of our Lord') are commonly used in texts in the English language to denote dates before and after the start of the Christian calendar.

**Figure 1.7** Expansion of the human population of the world from 40 000 BC to AD 2025. The diameter of each ring corresponds to the estimated population number at that date. (Source: data derived from McEvedy and Jones, 1978)

### 1.2.4 The human impact on planet Earth

No discussion of the nature of the environment in which humans live today can ignore the fact that planet Earth is facing an unprecedented environmental crisis. We have space here for just a brief summary of the major components:

1   Humans are destroying the Earth's natural resources. The world's coal, oil and natural gas supplies are being used up and its forests and wilderness areas are being destroyed. There is a chronic shortage of clean freshwater in many parts of the world.

2   The number of animal and plant species becoming extinct over recent decades is between 1000 and 10 000 times greater than scientists predict would be occurring naturally (Pimm et al., 1995). Box 1.1 gives an example.

3   Humans generate an enormous number of toxic (poisonous) substances, which are released into the environment. Major sources are smoke containing carbon dioxide and other gases from power plants, factories, vehicles and aircraft; the pesticides, herbicides and fertilisers used in intensive agriculture; and other chemical pollutants from industrial processes.

4   The spread of infectious, disease-causing organisms around the world (e.g. cholera) and the emergence of new ones (e.g. HIV/AIDS).

The impact of all the above factors is amplified by the continuing expansion of the human population (Figure 1.7). You will look more closely at factors 1, 3 and 4 in Chapter 3 of this book, which discusses the effects on human health of deteriorating water quality worldwide. In the past, environmental change was seen as a localised phenomenon; the world could be separated into areas where people lived, areas of agriculture and protected areas where wildlife could be conserved. Climate change alters all that. A majority of scientists now recognises that, for example, driving a large, 'gas-guzzling' car does not simply pollute the air in its immediate neighbourhood, but also contributes to global changes in the weather. The realisation that the natural environment is being affected on a global scale has forced a fundamental change in the way the natural world is viewed.

---

**Box 1.1** (Enrichment) **The global decline among the world's amphibians**

A major effort is being made to determine the conservation status of the world's amphibians (frogs, toads, newts and salamanders) (AmphibiaWeb, 2007; Global Amphibian Assessment, 2007). By September 2006, a total of 6084 species had been described and named (this figure increases by one or two species each week). Of these, 165 were thought to have become extinct in the previous 25 years. Some of these extinctions occurred in supposedly protected areas, such as national parks. Forty-three per cent of species were in decline and 1896 species (32%) were categorised as being threatened with extinction. The causes of amphibian declines are complex; most reflect a degradation in the Earth's freshwater habitats.

---

Natural habitats and their animal and plant inhabitants can no longer be conserved simply by creating national parks, nature reserves and 'green belts', because climate change and pollution affect them too. The most obvious symptom of the environmental crisis is a loss of **biodiversity** of plants and animals at a rate that is currently greater than at any time in the Earth's history. 'Biodiversity' is a word that has no single standard definition; it refers to both the number of species in a locality, region or the whole planet, and the number in the population of each species. The rapid decline in biodiversity is occurring not only in areas directly destroyed by human development, but also in supposedly protected areas. Putting a fence around biodiversity is not protecting it. So what? Why does it matter if tigers, or gorillas, or orchids, disappear?

It matters because habitat destruction and pollution have not only local, but global effects, partly through climate change. This is of great relevance to the study of human sciences because global climate change has a major impact on human health. For example, the thinning of the ozone layer in the Earth's atmosphere (Figure 1.8) that protects the Earth from ultraviolet radiation has caused a dramatic rise in the incidence of skin cancer in many parts of the world. In 2000, approximately 60 000 people died worldwide from excessive exposure to ultraviolet radiation (Lucas et al., 2006). Based on current trends, children could be three times more likely than their grandparents to develop malignant melanoma, a cancer that arises from the pigmented cells in the skin (Cancer Research UK, 2007). As discussed in Chapter 3, water, a natural resource vital to human health, is being exploited and polluted on a global scale, with dire consequences for the Earth's natural inhabitants and for its people.

The causes of some declines and extinctions among animals and plants are very obvious; tigers, for example, are close to extinction because of destruction of their habitat and from hunting. For other organisms, however, including many of the amphibians described in Box 1.1, declines and extinctions are described as 'enigmatic', meaning that no obvious cause is apparent. A reason to be concerned

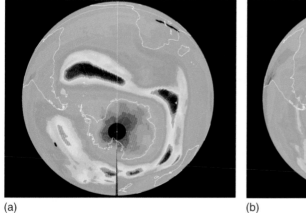
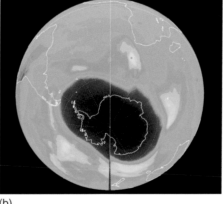

(a)　　　　　　　　　　　　　　　　(b)

**Figure 1.8** The ozone hole over the Antarctic, photographed on (a) 24 September 1980, and (b) on 8 October 2006 from a NASA satellite. In 2006, the hole covers the whole of Antarctica and extends to the tip of South America. Purple and black show where the ozone layer is thinnest, red where it is thickest. (Photo: Ozone Processing Team at NASA's Goddard Space Flight Center)

about them is that they may be providing early warning of environmental changes that, if left unchecked, will threaten other forms of life, including people. They are like 'canaries in a coal mine'. Coal miners used to take canaries with them into coal mines; more sensitive than humans to poisonous gases, they provided a living early-warning system. If the canary lost consciousness, the miners quickly evacuated the area. Population declines among the world's amphibians may be an early warning of an environmental catastrophe to come (Halliday, 2000).

Climate change is also having an immediate impact on human health. Over two weeks in the summer of 2003, as many as 45 000 people, mostly elderly, are thought to have died of over-heating in Europe; globally, the WHO estimates that climate change costs 150 thousand lives annually (Patz et al., 2005). It is also expected to have a variety of less direct effects on human health and well-being.

◆ Can you suggest some examples?

◆ They include an increase in the frequency and severity of extreme weather events such as hurricanes and tidal waves, which kill, disable and displace many thousands and destroy homes, agricultural land and livelihoods; malnutrition and famine due to crop failures and the death of livestock caused by prolonged droughts in some regions and flooding in others; and the spread of infectious diseases in refugee camps, in malnourished populations and where flooding causes mass contamination of drinking water.

Importantly, the health burden of these effects will not be shared equally across the world (Epstein, 2005; Foley et al., 2005; Kalkstein and Smoyer, 1993; Schiermeier, 2005).

> Climate change represents one of the greatest environmental and health equity challenges of our times; wealthy energy consuming nations are most responsible for global warming, yet poor countries are most at risk.
>
> (Patz and Kovats, 2002)

Demonstrating that 'poor countries' – and indeed disadvantaged people everywhere – are most at risk requires the comparison of health data from different countries. But this is not a straightforward matter, and we must make a brief diversion to explain why.

## 1.2.5 Classifying countries

Throughout this book (and others in this series) you will often see countries referred to as either 'developed' or 'developing', grouping all the nations of the world into these two broad categories. These terms are in widespread use in speeches and publications by the UN, the WHO, and governments, charities and voluntary organisations all over the world. Classifying countries in this way helps to illuminate the sharply differing health experiences of richer and poorer nations, but it also creates several problems.

There is no dispute about the *general* features of so-called **developed countries**: they provide universal education for their children; their populations have high rates of literacy; they have comprehensive high-technology health services (Figure 1.9); and they meet certain other development indicators, such as 100% access to safe drinking water and sanitation. Their economies grew rapidly in the early 20th century as a result of industrialisation, and they include all the richest nations on Earth.

However, there is considerable variation between international agencies about *which* countries are included in the 'developed' category. The World Bank uses a system based solely on the annual income generated per capita (per 'head' of population). If it exceeds an arbitrary threshold (revised each year), then a country is considered to be 'developed'. In 2003 the threshold for developed economies was just over US$ 10 000 per person. (The World Bank expresses each nation's wealth in US dollars (US$) so that comparisons can be made between countries.)

The United Nations uses a different system that includes income, but emphasises other development indicators such as health and participation rates in education. In 2003 the UN included 27 countries in its 'developed economy' classification: all of Western Europe and North America, Australia and Japan, the countries shown in cream in Figure 1.10. The UN excluded the former communist countries of Eastern Europe and put them into a separate category called 'transitional economies' (purple in Figure 1.10), a decision based on political history rather than on wealth or development. However, most of the health data identified as from developed

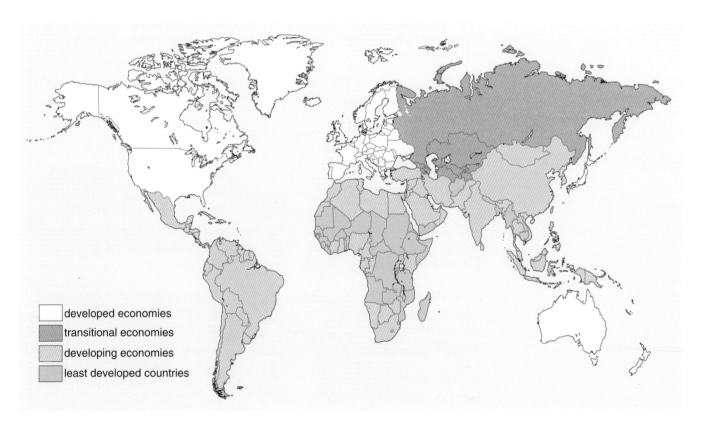

**Figure 1.9**   Health scientists in a hospital pathology laboratory in England. (Photo: Mike Levers/Open University)

- developed economies
- transitional economies
- developing economies
- least developed countries

**Figure 1.10**   The United Nations groups countries into four categories. In 2003 they classified 27 as 'developed economies' (cream), 27 'transitional economies' (purple), 88 'developing economies' (orange), and 50 'least developed countries' (green). (Source: United Nations, 2003)

*countries* that you will see in this book (including those from the WHO) come from *combining* the UN's developed and transitional economies. Just to confuse matters the WHO sometimes uses the narrower UN 'developed economy' classification, and we will take care to point out when this happens.

The remaining countries shown in Figure 1.10 are only partly industrialised and their national wealth is below that of the developed economies. They rely to a much greater degree on agriculture, small industrial businesses and low-paid unskilled or low-skilled labour. Major indicators of development, such as literacy and provision of clean water vary hugely between these countries, yet they are generally grouped together as **developing countries** in most sources of health data. However, you may encounter UN data which distinguishes those that are undergoing rapid economic development, the 'developing economies' of South and Central America, South East Asia and some parts of Africa (orange in Figure 1.10), and the 'least developed countries' (or LDCs; green in Figure 1.10), which include Afghanistan, Bangladesh and most of sub-Saharan Africa. In 2003, the national wealth of the LDCs was less than US$ 800 per capita, which translates into an average of just over US$ 2 per person per day.

To give you some idea of the health impact on people living in countries with such widely divergent development status, the average life expectancy in 2002 in Sierra Leone (an LDC) was just 34 years; in the United Kingdom it was 78. (We will discuss life expectancy further in Section 1.4.1.) However, beware of assuming that there is a neat correspondence between national wealth and longevity; also in 2002, life expectancy in Bangladesh (another LDC) was 61 years. You will explore some of the reasons for such striking disparities later in this chapter.

So, to sum up, many (but not all) sources of international health data combine the UN's developed and transitional economies under the label *developed countries*, and they combine the UN's developing economies and least developed countries under the label *developing countries*. However, any classification that groups all the countries of the world into two (or even the UN's four) categories may hide more than it reveals about the factors that shape the health of different populations.

◆ Can you suggest why?

◆ There must be significant health differences between countries in the *same* category, but these could be disguised by lumping together the health data from all 'developed' and all 'developing' countries.

For example, China, India and Zimbabwe were all classified as 'developing economies' by the UN in 2003. But China and India have rapid economic growth and their life expectancy and child health indicators are improving, whereas the Zimbabwean economy is in steep decline, along with the health of its people.

A further problem is that there is a wide range of health experience *within* every country. To refer to a country as 'developed' or 'developing' disguises the fact that there are rich and poor in every population. Individual social and economic circumstances are a stronger influence on a person's health than their country's classification. For example, comparisons of the **infant mortality rate** or **IMR** of different populations reveals striking inequalities within some countries.

The IMR is an internationally recognised health indicator and refers to the number of babies in every 1000 live births who die in their first year of life. In South Africa (one of the UN's 'developing economies'), the IMR for white babies in 2002 was around 7 infant deaths per 1000 live births; for black babies it was close to 50 per 1000. This has a major influence on average life expectancy (Figure 1.11). You should be aware of issues like these when you study the health data presented later in this book.

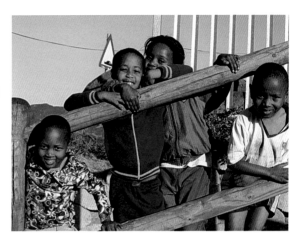

**Figure 1.11** The average life expectancy of these South African children is estimated to be at least 20 years less than that of their white counterparts. (Photo: Jeroen Daniel Kraan (Holland)/Flickr Photo Sharing)

### 1.2.6 Megacities

We can now return to the theme of the 'human zoo' and its effects on health. In 1975, there were four cities in the world with a population exceeding ten million people: Tokyo, New York, Shanghai and Mexico City. In 2003, there were 20 as shown in the **bar chart** in Figure 1.12. (If you are unfamiliar with 'reading' bar charts, see Box 1.2.)

---

**Box 1.2** (Explanation) Reading a bar chart

A bar chart is a simple way of presenting numerical data visually, so as to emphasise the relative size of different numbers. In the example below, the bars are stacked *horizontally* with the longest at the top and the shortest at the bottom, but bar charts can also be drawn with *vertical* bars (as in Figures 1.22 and 1.24 later in this book). In Figure 1.12, Tokyo has a population of 35 million, which is nearly twice that of Mexico City, with 18.7 million, so the bar for Tokyo is nearly twice the length of the bar for Mexico City.

---

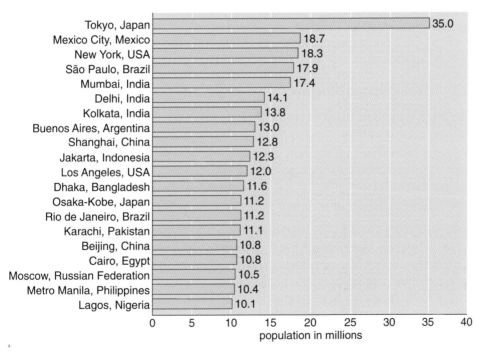

**Figure 1.12** Bar chart showing megacities with more than 10 million inhabitants in 2003. (Source: Marshall, 2005, p. 313)

◆ Compare Figure 1.12 with Figure 1.10. How many of the 20 megacities in Figure 1.12 are *outside* the 'developed economies' (cream) in Figure 1.10? What are the exceptions?

◆ Sixteen of the megacities are not in the developed economies. The four exceptions are New York and Los Angeles in the USA, and Tokyo and Osaka-Kobe in Japan.

Dhaka, in Bangladesh, is the fastest growing megacity and is in one of the world's poorest countries. Jakarta in Indonesia is another rapidly growing megacity. It had a population of 12.3 million people in 2003; by 2015 this is expected to rise to 17.5 million. As in many large cities, air pollution is a major health hazard in Jakarta. Respiratory diseases account for 12.6% of deaths in Jakarta and there are over one million asthma attacks annually. Water and sanitation are also major problems. Only 60% of Jakarta's population has access to a piped supply of water and even that is so polluted it has to be boiled before consumption. Only 3% of sewage finds its way to a sewage plant; most goes into inadequate, leaking septic tanks or into open water, along with a huge amount of domestic rubbish (Figure 1.13). As in many megacities, a large proportion of the population lives in shanty towns, where health problems are particularly severe.

Conditions in Jakarta are mirrored in many of the world's largest cities, which tend to have high levels of violence and traffic-related injuries. In Manila, three out of every four people live in unauthorised housing in shanty towns. In Mexico City, air pollution contributes to 6400 deaths every year and 29% of children have unhealthy levels of lead in their blood (Marshall, 2005). You will look further at the health problems due to pollution in large cities in Chapter 3. The urban environment of today is very different from the conditions in which humans evolved and this has implications for human health, as you will see next.

## 1.3 A very short history of human evolution

Nothing in biology makes sense except in the light of evolution.

(Theodosius Dobzhansky, 1973)

### 1.3.1 Biological evolution

The word 'evolution' simply means 'change over time'. The motor car has evolved since it was first invented; cars are faster, more comfortable, more reliable and more fuel-efficient than their 'ancestors' of many years ago. Car evolution is a result of technological change and is a very different process from biological evolution, which has resulted in living plants and animals being different from their ancestors, the nature of which is known from fossilised remains.

Biologists often consider the evolution of specific features or 'characteristics' of plants or animals. A characteristic of great interest in the evolution of humans is brain size, which has increased dramatically during human evolution. An ancestor of modern humans, *Australopithecus africanus* (see Box 1.3), lived in Africa 2.5 million years ago and had a brain volume of 400 cm³; modern humans have a brain volume of about 1360 cm³, an increase of 340% (Lewin, 1999). How has such a dramatic change occurred?

Respiratory disease is discussed in another book in this series *Chronic Obstructive Pulmonary Disease: A Forgotten Killer* (Midgley, 2008).

Traffic accidents and violence are discussed in another book in this series, *Trauma, Repair and Recovery* (Phillips, 2008).

 If you are studying this book as part of an Open University course, now would be a good time to undertake Activity C1 in the *Companion*.

A cubic centimetre (cm³) is the volume of a cube with sides each of 1 centimetre.

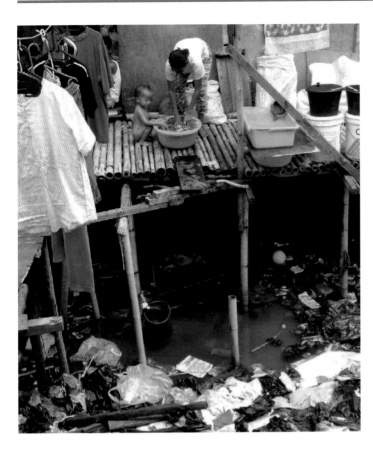

**Figure 1.13** Kampung Kandang shanty town, Jakarta, Indonesia. A woman is washing her clothes in a bucket that will be emptied into the rubbish-strewn water below. (Source: Marshall, 2005, p. 314)

---

**Box 1.3** (Explanation) How organisms are named in biology

*Australopithecus africanus* provides an example of how organisms are named in biology. This naming system uses two Latin or Greek words, the first referring to a number of similar species, the second to one specific species. At least six species of *Australopithecus* have been described. *Australopithecus robustus* was a species with particularly large teeth. Species names are always printed in italics and are often abbreviated, as in *A. africanus*.

---

A common error in discussions of biological evolution is to argue that a characteristic such as a large brain evolved because it is 'good for the species'. While it may seem obvious that having a larger brain would make a species more intelligent, and therefore more successful, the process that drives biological evolution, **natural selection**, does not work that way. Natural selection is a process that arises inevitably if there are differences between individuals within a species (in other words, there is *variation*). As in modern humans, some individuals among human ancestors had larger brains, some smaller. If having a larger brain confers an advantage on an individual in terms of having an advantage over other members *of the same species* in the struggle to survive and reproduce, it will leave more offspring in the next generation than will individuals with smaller brains. A characteristic that gives an individual such an advantage is said to be **adaptive**. This will lead to evolutionary change over many generations, provided a crucial condition is met, namely that variation in brain size is determined, at least in part, by *genes*. A characteristic that does not have a genetic basis will not evolve through natural selection. For example, a person who, during their life, develops a particularly muscular physique will not pass that physique on to their children.

Natural selection will thus bring about change in a characteristic, from one generation to the next, if three conditions exist: (i) the characteristic must show variation, (ii) such variation must have a genetic basis, (iii) such variation must lead to variation in reproductive success (i.e. it must be adaptive). Condition (iii) will exist if there is competition between individuals for the environmental resources required to survive and reproduce. This is generally true; in most species far more offspring are produced than can survive to reproduce.

Biological evolution, brought about by natural selection, occurs by small changes occurring from one generation to the next. There are no 'great leaps forward' as there can be in technological evolution; a sudden, radical transition, like that from propeller-driven to jet-powered aircraft, does not occur by natural selection. Because biological evolution occurs in small steps, it is generally assumed to be a slow process; it took 2.5 million years for the human brain to treble in size. The speed of biological evolution varies from one species to another and depends on its generation time. Generation time is the average time interval between an individual's birth and the birth of its children; in humans, the generation time is about 20 years. In many plants and animals, generation time is much shorter (a year in annual plants and many animals) and it follows that, in such species, the rate of evolution can be quite fast. As a result, there are many examples of plants and animals that have undergone evolutionary change within recorded history. For example, several roadside plants have evolved the ability to withstand the effect of salt spread on roads in winter; the mosquitoes that carry malaria have evolved resistance to many of the insecticides that have been used to control them.

Of particular relevance to this book, the generation time of bacteria (and other microscopic agents), including those that cause disease, is very short indeed. In some bacteria, generation time can be as short as 12 minutes; in others it can be a few days. The very short generation time of bacteria means that they can evolve very rapidly in comparison with slow-reproducing species such as humans. In one hour, a bacterial species can complete five generations; it takes humans 100 years to do so. This means that the bacteria that live in our bodies are evolving in our lifetime, and are adapting to whatever defences our bodies make against them. Most importantly, bacteria can very rapidly evolve resistance to antibiotics, a topic that is discussed in detail later in this chapter (Activity 1.1 Antibiotics and bacterial growth).

### 1.3.2 Human evolution

Megacities and shanty towns are a very recent feature of human evolution but, in most aspects of their biology, their human inhabitants have not changed since humans were hunter-gatherers living in the African savannah. This section looks, very briefly, at the evolution of humans and draws attention to certain aspects of human biology that are a 'legacy' of ancient human ancestry.

Humans belong to a group of **mammals** called the primates (Figure 1.14). Humans share a number of characteristics with other mammals, notably hair and feeding infants on breast milk. The **primates**, a group that includes humans,

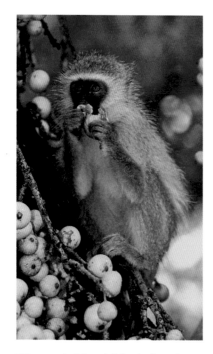

**Figure 1.14** A black-faced vervet monkey (*Cercopithecus aethiops*) eating fruit in a tree. Like most other primates, vervet monkeys are arboreal and have hands that can manipulate small objects. (Tony Camacho/Science Photo Library)

lemurs, monkeys and apes, have a large brain, well-developed eyes and hands that can grasp and manipulate objects. Most primates are arboreal (tree-dwelling) and are confined to woodland and forest. Between 1.8 and 3.0 million years ago, global climate change led to a drier climate across Africa; much of the forest disappeared to be replaced by savannah grassland. Baboons, and the ancestors of humans, the **hominids**, adapted to this new habitat. They became adept at moving fast over an open landscape in which there were many predators. It is generally believed that early hominids, like present-day baboons, lived in tight-knit, cohesive social groups that enhanced their ability to detect and defend themselves against predators and to locate dispersed sources of food. (Ideas about early human evolution are essentially speculative. The evidence comes from a very limited number of fossilised bones and teeth and from comparisons with living animals, such as baboons, that live in a habitat similar to that of our human ancestors.)

Primates are essentially vegetarian, eating leaves and fruits, though many species occasionally kill and eat other animals. It is clear from the fossilised teeth of early hominids that they were *omnivorous*, that is, eating both plant and animal food. Living in groups enabled them to hunt and eat animals much larger than themselves. It is likely that they also fed on animals killed by specialist carnivores (meat-eaters) such as lions.

At some point in their evolution (the date is disputed, but at least 500 000 years ago), hominids acquired the ability to control fires and so were able to cook their food. This development is reflected in ancestral human teeth, and to some extent in modern dental health. Eating raw foods, particularly abrasive leaves, coarse roots and nuts, requires a lot of chewing and the fossilised teeth of early hominids and present-day hunter-gatherers are notably scoured and worn down. They show little evidence of tooth decay, however.

◆ What effect on dental health do you think occurred when settled agricultural communities replaced the nomadic way of life? (Figure 1.15 contains a clue.)

◆ The ability to grind and cook cereal crops and vegetables rendered them soft enough to eat, but these foods are rich in sticky carbohydrates which form a coating on the teeth. (Modern diets in developed countries also contain large quantities of refined sugars.) Bacteria in the mouth thrive in this habitat and attack the enamel surface of the teeth, causing gum disease and tooth decay.

Unlike baboons, humans evolved an upright posture called **bipedality** (bye-peed-al-itee), walking and running on their hind legs. Bipedal posture has many advantages; it enables humans to see further and it frees the arms for carrying and manipulating objects. It involved many changes in the skeleton in comparison with the modern apes, the closest relatives of humans (Figure 1.16, overleaf). But being upright puts great strain on the hip joints and the high frequency of hip problems in elderly people may be a legacy of the evolution of bipedality. Despite four million years of walking upright, humans today have a backbone that, under the strain of carrying the full weight of the trunk and head, is prone to injury. The human backbone is a compromise between strength and flexibility, between a structure that will carry

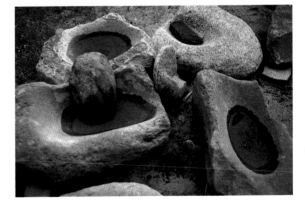

**Figure 1.15** Grinding tools at Little Petra, Jordan, where agriculture was well established 8000 years ago. Grain was ground in the hollowed-out bowls by a person pushing and pulling a hard rounded stone backwards and forwards. (Photo: Caroline Pond)

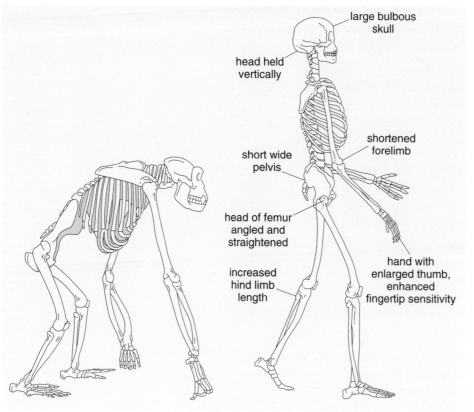

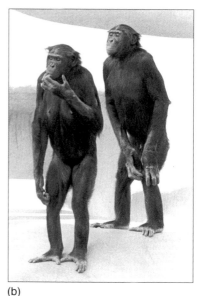

(b)

(a)

**Figure 1.16**   Ape and human anatomy compared. (a) The evolution of bipedality in humans involved a number of changes in the skeleton. (b) All apes can stand upright, but even these bonobo chimpanzees (*Pan paniscus*), whose erect posture is closest to that of humans, cannot walk far on two legs. (Source: Lewin, 1999, p. 81; Photo: Dr Franz B. M. De Waal)

weight in all circumstances and one that allows a person to run, or throw a spear. In the contemporary industrialised world, more working days are lost through back pain and back injury than from any other cause (Dunbar and Barrett, 2000).

To run fast on two legs requires a more compact pelvis than running on four legs. Modern women have a wider pelvis than men, which contributes to the fact that they cannot run quite as fast. A feature of hominid evolution is an enormous increase in the size of the brain compared with ancestral primates, which is why human babies need a wide birth canal and women have a broad pelvis. Most primates give birth when the infant's brain has developed to its full size, but human babies are born long before this. If a baby stayed in the womb until its brain reached adult size, pregnancy would last 21 months (Dunbar, 2004) and the adult female pelvis would have to be so wide that speed and mobility would be greatly reduced.

◆   What effect would this have had on the survival of the human species?

◆   There would have been lower survival rates among ancestral females because they would have been less able to escape from predators, and this in turn would have led to fewer births among females with longer pregnancies.

So the modern human pelvis represents a compromise between two opposing pressures: the need for speed and the need to give birth. This is an example of what is known as an **evolutionary-trade-off**: evolution cannot produce a perfectly adapted human body because 'trade-offs' have to be made between competing demands.

There has also been a trade-off in infant development. Babies are safer in the womb than in the outside world, favouring a long pregnancy, but a large brain requires an early birth, or a very wide pelvis. By comparison with animals like baboons, whose babies can run around very soon after birth, human babies are totally dependent on parental care for many months after birth. These trade-offs may also account for the fact that childbirth appears to be more painful in humans than in other primates. It may also contribute to the high mortality around birth, in both infant and mother, which occurred until very recently in developed countries, and remains so in many developing countries. Of course, other factors are involved, for example the availability of trained birth-care attendants, but our descent from hominids who had to 'run for their lives' should not be discounted.

## 1.4 Costs and benefits of life in developed countries

These are strange times, when we are healthier than ever but more anxious about our health.

(Professor Roy Porter, medical historian, 1997)

Accurate statistics on the causes of death, disease and disability do not go back very far into human history, but it is clear that nowadays most people die for very different reasons than they did in the not-so-distant past. Some causes of injuries and death have been almost completely eliminated in developed countries, such as attack by predators, which still claim thousands of lives in rural areas of the developing world. Other hazards have been introduced, notably traffic accidents, which kill or permanently disable over 5 million people worldwide every year.

Another book in this series (Phillips, 2008) deals with traffic-related accidents in more detail.

### 1.4.1 Increasing life expectancy

Changes in human health over time are often represented by a **proxy measure** (a readily measurable statistic that 'stands in' for something more complex), for example, the infant mortality rate (or IMR; Section 1.2.4). Another commonly used proxy measure is *life expectancy* (also known as longevity), which is an estimate of the *average* length of life from birth to death of everyone in a particular population. Life expectancy has been rising everywhere since the mid-19th century, except in countries badly affected by HIV/AIDS, where it has been falling since around 1990, and among Russian men, where alcohol poisoning is a growing cause of death.

The impact of alcohol poisoning in Russia is discussed in another book in this series, *Alcohol and Human Health* (Smart, 2007).

A typical woman in the UK in 2004 could expect to live to 81 years, an average of 6 years more than her counterpart in 1970, and 32 years longer than British women in 1901 (UK National Statistics, 2007), and double her life expectancy in 1837 (Porter, 1997). Much of the improvement in longevity worldwide is due to a substantial reduction in mortality among children under 1 year of age (infant mortality), which in the UK in 2000 was down to 5 deaths in every 1000 live births. Maternal mortality associated with childbirth has also declined. In some 19th-century maternity hospitals in England, between 9 and 10% of women entering died; in 1930, an English woman had a 1 in 250 chance of not surviving labour (Porter, 1997); by 2000, the risk of dying during childbirth was down to 13 deaths per 100 000 births (UN Millennium Development Goals, 2005).

While the reliability of statistical data falls rapidly the further back one goes in time, and there are limitations in the data-collection systems of even the richest countries, it is possible to find comparable data that shed light on the relative health of different populations. For example, Figure 1.17 shows the estimated life expectancy in the 30 countries belonging to the OECD in 1960 and 2002/2003.

The Organisation of Economic Cooperation and Development (OECD) is a confederation of 30 countries, committed to 'democratic government and market economics', which publishes reports and statistics on a range of economic and social issues, including health, science and innovation.

◆ In 2002/2003, which of the OECD countries in Figure 1.17 had the longest, and which the shortest, life expectancy?

◆ Of these countries, Japan had the longest, at 81.8 years; Turkey had the shortest, at 68.7 years.

◆ What was the general direction of change in life expectancy across all the countries in Figure 1.17 between 1960 and 2002/2003?

◆ It increased in every country, and the OECD average rose from 68.5 years in 1960 to 77.8 years in 2002/2003, an increase of 9.3 years. Note that countries with the shortest life expectancy in 1960 (e.g. Korea, Mexico, Turkey) increased by the largest amount.

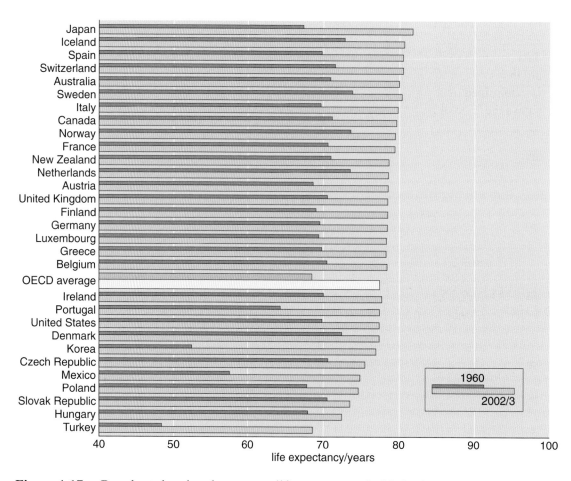

**Figure 1.17**   Bar chart showing the average life expectancy in 30 OECD countries, in 1960 and 2002/2003 (both sexes combined). The bars labelled 'OECD average' show life expectancy averaged across all 30 countries. (Source: OECD, 2005, p. 19)

These data show that, at least in OECD countries, life expectancy has increased substantially over a short period of recent human history. They also show that there are very considerable differences in life expectancy between even this relatively high-income group of countries. The differences are much greater between the richest and poorest countries in the world. To investigate why this is, an obvious first step is to see how data on life expectancy are related, across the 30 countries, to some measure of their prosperity. Figure 1.18 is a **scatter plot** showing such an analysis, using a measure of the amount of money spent in each country on providing health services. If you are unfamiliar with 'reading' scatter plots, study Box 1.4 and Figure 1.18.

---

**Box 1.4** (Explanation) Interpreting a scatter plot

A scatter plot is a way of showing whether two numerical *variables* are related (in Figure 1.18 they are 'health spending per capita' and 'life expectancy'). They are called 'variables' because they can each have a range of possible values. Each *data point* on this scatter plot represents a particular country; for example, Turkey (TUR) spent about US$ 500 per capita on health in 2003, and its people had an average life expectancy of 68.7 years. The pattern in the data points shows whether or not there is an *association* between the two variables. If you now look at the spread of data points in Figure 1.18, you can see that they are roughly arranged in an arc that slopes upwards from left to right. The curved line in Figure 1.18 is determined by a mathematical procedure that need not concern you; it shows the 'line of best fit' through the 30 data points.

---

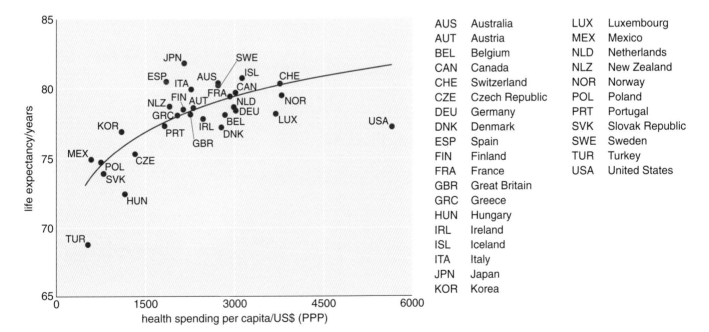

**Figure 1.18**   Scatter plot showing average life expectancy in 2003 in OECD countries in relation to health expenditure per capita in US dollars (converted to 'purchasing power parities' or PPP, a measure that takes into account differences in how much a dollar can purchase in each country). (Source: OECD, 2005, p. 19)

Note in Figure 1.18 that the point for Great Britain (GBR is the international standard abbreviation for the whole United Kingdom, i.e. England, Wales, Scotland and Northern Ireland) is on the line. This means that life expectancy in Great Britain is exactly what you would expect, on average, for a country with Britain's level of health spending, based on the overall pattern across these 30 countries. Notice that countries falling well *above* the 'best fit' line, such as Japan (JPN) and Spain (ESP), have *better* than average life expectancy than you would expect from their health expenditure.

◆ What is the relationship between life expectancy and health spending in countries that fall *below* the line, such as the USA and Hungary (HUN)?

◆ Life expectancy in these countries is *lower* than average, relative to the amount they spend on their health services.

◆ Do the data presented in Figure 1.18 suggest that spending on health is *positively* associated with life expectancy (i.e. when one is high, so is the other)?

◆ Yes, they do. There is a lot of scatter in the data but, in general, countries such as Mexico (MEX), Poland (POL) and the Slovak Republic (SVK), which had relatively low health spending in 2003, also had lower than average life expectancy for an OECD country; those with high spending, such as Iceland (ISL), Switzerland (CHE) and Norway (NOR) also had higher than average life expectancy.

However, there are many exceptions to the *general* pattern shown in Figure 1.18; for example, health spending per capita in Japan was less than half that in the USA in 2003, yet Japan had the higher life expectancy by about five years. There are many reasons why an overall measure of health expenditure does not correlate precisely with life expectancy, or with any other 'proxy measure' of a nation's health. One is that the health budget includes expenditure on many different aspects of health provision, only some of which have a direct impact on life expectancy. Furthermore, life expectancy is only a proxy measure of 'health status' and cannot reflect all the various dimensions of health, disease and disability in a population. As well as the total amount spent on health, it is important to consider how that expenditure is distributed *within* each population. Inequalities in access to health services partly explain the discrepancy in longevity between Japan and the USA. Resources for health are distributed reasonably equitably in Japan (Figure 1.19), whereas in the USA there is a substantial 'under-class' that receives poor health care and has lower than average life expectancy for a country with that level of wealth.

## 1.4.2 Decreasing child mortality

A major benefit of living in a developed country is a low level of child mortality, a factor that contributes substantially to higher life expectancy. Figure 1.20 shows how the infant mortality rate (IMR) has changed in the recent

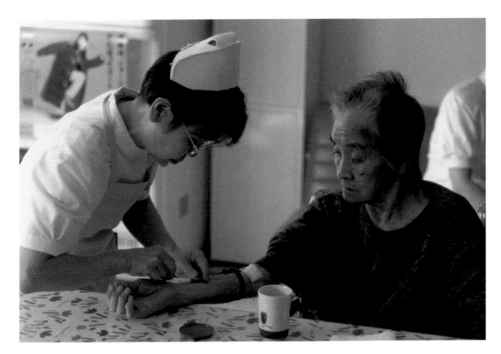

**Figure 1.19** High-quality health care in Japan reaches the whole population, which partly explains why Japanese life expectancy is the highest in the world. (Photo: Mark Henley/Panos Pictures)

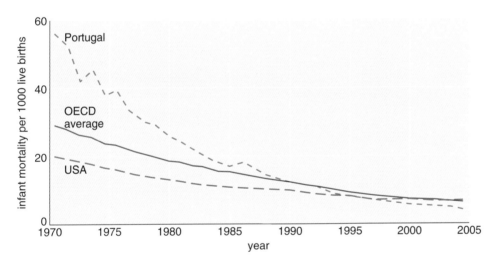

**Figure 1.20** Line graph showing changes in the infant mortality rate in Portugal, USA and the OECD average, 1970 to 2003. (Source: OECD, 2005, p. 31)

past in two OECD countries, Portugal and the USA, compared with the average for all 30 OECD countries combined. As you can see, small improvements in this proxy measure of human health are still being made even in the world's most developed countries. The situation with regards to child mortality is very different in developing countries.

**Table 1.1** Child mortality rate (deaths under 5 years per 1000 live births) in 20 countries in 2003 selected according to their development status (as given in Figure 1.10). (Source: data derived from WHO, 2005a, Table 1)

| Least developed countries | Developing economies | Transitional economies | Developed economies |
|---|---|---|---|
| 283 – Sierra-Leone | 87 – India | 16 – Russian Federation | 8 – USA |
| 260 – Angola | 41 – Algeria | 15 – Bulgaria | 6 – Australia |
| 257 – Afghanistan | 39 – Egypt | 14 – Serbia-Montenegro | 6 – United Kingdom |
| 82 – Nepal | 38 – Nicaragua | 8 – Poland | 5 – France |
| 69 – Bangladesh | 37 – China | 5 – Czech Republic | 4 – Japan |

Table 1.1 shows the child mortality rates in 2003 for 20 countries, five in each of the four development categories explained in Figure 1.10, selected to illustrate the inequalities in this proxy measure of health. The **child mortality rate** is the number of children who die under five years of age in a given year, expressed per 1000 live births.

◆ How would you describe the relationship, across all 20 countries, between development status and child mortality rates?

◆ In general, the more 'developed' a country's economy is, the lower is its child mortality rate.

◆ What do you notice about the *variation* in child mortality between countries within the same development category?

◆ Variation in the mortality rate is very high in the least developed countries, ranging from 69 to 283 children in every 1000 births who die before their fifth birthday. The range is smaller in the developing economies (from 37 to 87), smaller still in the former communist transitional economies (from 5 to 16), and least of all in the developed economies (from 4 to 8).

Child mortality is much lower in some developing countries such as Bangladesh than in others, largely because children have benefited from targeted immunisation and nutritional programmes.

### 1.4.3 Increasing human mobility

One of the most dramatic changes that has occurred in the life of humans in recent times is an increase in mobility, especially among people living in affluent countries. The development of road, rail and air transport has enabled people to travel much further and more often in the course of their lives than they could just a few generations ago (Figure 1.21).

Increased mobility brings enormous benefits, but it also inflicts serious costs on society, including atmospheric pollution that contributes to climate change, and

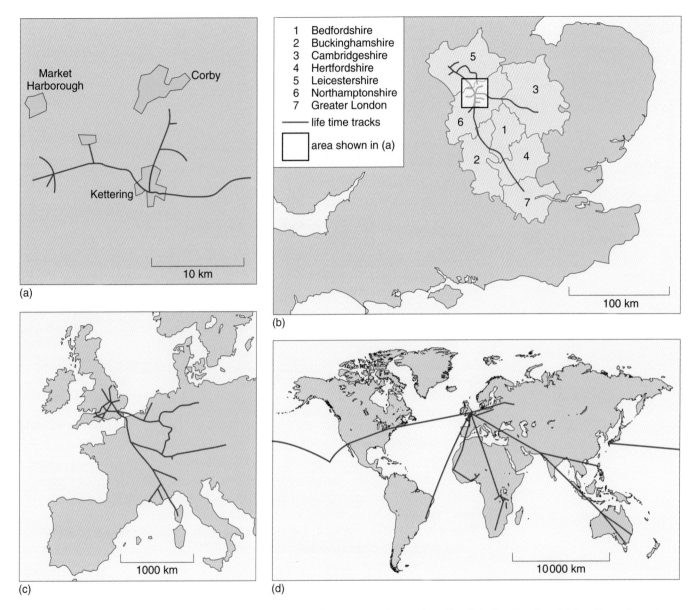

**Figure 1.21** Maps showing changing mobility over four generations of an English family. David Bradley plotted the lifetime travel of (a) his great-grandfather, (b) his grandfather, (c) his father and (d) himself. (Source: Cliff and Haggett, 2004, p. 91)

the spread of infectious diseases around the world. For example, cholera, a disease you will read about in Chapter 3, was originally confined to Asia, but in the last 40 years it has become globally prevalent. An outbreak of an infectious disease in a community, region or country that involves a large number of people is called an **epidemic**. If cases spread on a worldwide scale, it is called a **pandemic**.

Currently, the world is experiencing what is called the seventh cholera pandemic. This began in Indonesia in 1961, not as a sudden increase in the number of people affected (see Figure 1.22, overleaf), but due to the appearance of a new form of the bacterium *Vibrio cholerae* (vib-ree-oh kol-er-eye), the O1, or El Tor strain, which causes the disease.

The terms 'epidemic' and 'pandemic' were originally applied only to infectious diseases; they are now often applied to non-infectious conditions (such as obesity) or health-damaging behaviours (such as drinking and driving) that seem to be rapidly increasing.

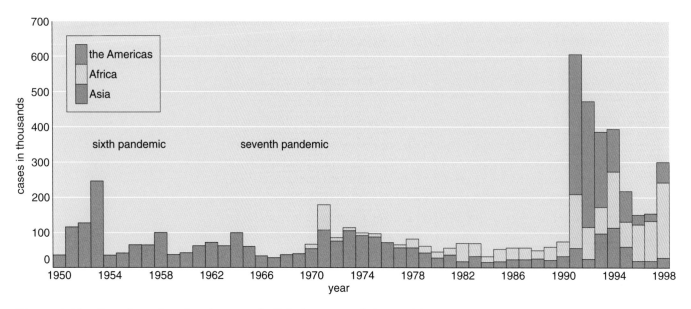

**Figure 1.22** Bar chart showing the spread of cholera around the world, 1950–1998. (Source: WHO, 2000, Figure 4.7, p. 3)

◆ Look at Figure 1.22. When did cholera first spread to Africa and when did it reach the Americas?

◆ It arrived in Africa in 1970 and in the Americas in 1991.

The arrival of cholera in South America illustrates the role of international transport in the spread of infectious disease. A ship from China discharged its bilges into the sea at Callao, the port for Lima in Peru, where conditions were ideal for the proliferation and spread of the cholera bacterium, which lives in shallow water. The accidental way in which infectious diseases can be spread from one part of the world to another has led to the development, as in the case of avian (bird) flu, of international collaborative efforts to monitor disease outbreaks and to try to contain them.

### 1.4.4 Other benefits and costs of life in developed countries

Living in a developed country brings many health *benefits* to people, such as:

- Water and food can be delivered to people hygienically, that is mostly free of harmful bacteria and other pathogens. Hygiene, especially in water supplies, has played a much greater role than medical intervention in controlling most infectious diseases in developed countries. As sanitation and water treatment improved during the late 19th and early 20th centuries in Western Europe and the USA, deaths from infection fell sharply and in most cases reached relatively low levels well before immunisations were introduced.

- Many childhood infectious diseases, such as polio, measles and diphtheria, are now almost completely prevented by adequate immunisation programmes. In the poorer communities of developing countries they kill or disable hundreds of thousands of children.

- If people do become infected with pathogenic bacteria they can usually be treated successfully with antibiotics.

- People with inherited or acquired physical defects can often have them corrected or alleviated by surgery, physiotherapy, or devices such as artificial limbs or spectacles.

- Contraceptives enable most people to determine when they will have children and how many they will have.

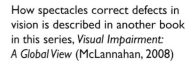

How spectacles correct defects in vision is described in another book in this series, *Visual Impairment: A Global View* (McLannahan, 2008)

Living in a developed country also carries certain health *costs*, including:

- People in towns and cities live close to one another and can encounter many hundreds of strangers in a single day, for example on crowded buses and trains (recall Figure 1.5). This makes it easier for infectious agents to spread from person to person.

- The environments created by human settlements can encourage the evolution of entirely new and harmful bacteria. An example is Legionnaires' disease, caused by *Legionella pneumophila* (leeja-nela new-mofila) bacteria, which seem to have evolved in the warm moist environment of air-conditioning systems in large buildings. It was named after the first outbreak in people attending a Legionnaires' convention at an American hotel.

- An enormous variety of chemicals manufactured for use in industry, agriculture and the home are released into the environment, some of which are harmful (see Chapter 3 of this book).

- The inappropriate and excessive use of antibiotics exerts **selection pressure** that promotes the evolution of new, antibiotic-resistant strains of bacteria. For example, *Staphylococcus aureus* (sta-fil-oh-cok-us or-ee-us) is a bacterium that is normally susceptible to methicillin (a penicillin-like antibiotic) and mainly causes skin rashes and abscesses. Methicillin-resistant *Staphylococcus aureus* (or MRSA) has evolved which can tolerate even the highest safe dose of methicillin that can be prescribed and is responsible for increasing numbers of severe wound infections in surgical wards and other hospital-acquired infections. Activity 1.1 demonstrates how **antibiotic resistance** can evolve more quickly when antibiotics are taken inappropriately.

## 1.4.5 Antibiotic resistance

## Activity I.I   Antibiotics and bacterial growth

Allow I hour

Now would be the ideal time to study the animation entitled 'Antibiotics and bacterial growth' on the DVD associated with this book. If you are unable to study it now, continue with the rest of the chapter and return to it as soon as you can.

In this activity you will learn how bacteria grow within a natural environment, the human gut, and about the effect of various doses of antibiotic on this process. By the end you should appreciate the importance of completing a course of antibiotics and how resistant strains can become more prevalent if antibiotics aren't taken correctly. The DVD includes interactive questions so you can self-assess your understanding.

Antibiotic resistance is not just a problem in developed countries; the greatest potential threat is the global spread of multi-drug resistant strains of *Mycobacterium tuberculosis* (my-koh-bak-teer-ee-um), the bacterium that causes TB. There are many other aspects of life in developed countries that could be added to the list of costs and benefits to health; you will look at two of them in the final two sections of this chapter.

## 1.5   Diet, obesity and the risk to health

One of the most dramatic current changes in human health worldwide is a massive increase in **obesity** (exceeding a certain threshold for body weight, taking height into account), and the health problems associated with it. Obesity can be regarded as a disease that has become a global epidemic, increasing in many developing as well as developed countries (Haslam and James, 2005). Current estimates suggest that being overweight now adversely affects more people in the world than does being under-nourished. Obesity provides a good illustration of how living in the 'human zoo' has created health problems that have their roots in the way humans adapted to their environment during their early evolution, as we will explain shortly.

While many people in the world are obese, many others have insufficient food and show stunted growth. **Stunting** is defined as being shorter at a given age by a specified amount below the population average. Both obesity and stunting are partly reflections of family income and, consequently, their occurrence across the world is related to the wealth of different countries (Figure 1.23).

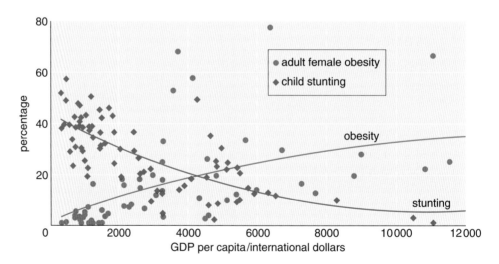

**Figure 1.23**   Scatter plot showing the level of stunting and obesity in different countries in relation to their national income. Stunting is given as the percentage of children under 5 years who are short for age; obesity is the percentage of females aged 15 years and over who are obese according to their body mass index (Box 5.1); national income is the gross domestic product (GDP) per capita, converted to standard 'international dollars'. Each point represents a different country and the curved lines are the lines of 'best fit' through the data points. (Source: WHO, 2006, chart 8, p. 17)

◆ Study Figure 1.23. (If you are unsure how to interpret a scatter plot with a 'best fit' line, go back and read Box 1.4 and the discussion of Figure 1.18 again). What is the relationship between stunting in children, obesity in adult females and the GDP of the countries shown?

◆ Stunting in children is more common in countries with low GDP, i.e. these two variables are *inversely* related; stunting is high when GDP is low and vice versa. By contrast, adult female obesity is *positively* related to GDP, i.e. when one is high, so is the other, and vice versa.

Note, however, that there are some widely scattered data points in Figure 1.23, indicating that the associations between these variables are not exact; there are significant numbers of obese adults in poorer countries and some stunted children even in the richest nations.

There are a number of different ways to determine whether a person is overweight or obese. The measure most often used is the **body mass index (BMI)** – Box 1.5.

---

**Box 1.5** (Explanation) Body mass index (BMI)

The BMI is calculated by dividing a person's weight (mass) in kilograms (kg) by their height in metres squared (m$^2$). A number squared is a number multiplied by itself; $3 \times 3$ can be written as $3^2$ (3 squared). The BMI of a person who is 1.7 m in height and weighs 65 kg is calculated as follows:

Height in metres squared = $1.7^2$ or $1.7 \times 1.7 = 2.89$

So BMI = $65 \div 2.89 = 22.49$

In most assessments based on BMI, people with a BMI of 20 to 24.9 are considered to be of normal healthy weight, those with a BMI of less than 20 are categorised as underweight, a BMI of 25 to 29.9 is said to be overweight, and greater than 30 is clinically obese. It is important to stress that such categorisations are arbitrary and that the thresholds have been changed from time to time. More importantly, they are very crude indices of health; it would be absurd simply to regard a person with a BMI of 24 as 'healthy' and a person with a BMI of 25 as 'unhealthy', for example.

---

Obesity is strongly associated with a number of health problems, including heart disease, high blood pressure, breast cancer, back pain, arthritis and diabetes. Having a BMI greater than 35 increases the risk of developing diabetes 93-fold in women and 42-fold in men (Jung, 1997). The increase in obesity has been especially rapid in China (Figure 1.24, overleaf). Using the WHO's criteria for calculating BMI, it has been estimated that, in 2002, 184 million Chinese people were overweight and 31 million were obese (Wu, 2006). This makes the point that obesity is not confined to the wealthy industrialised countries.

GDP is a measure of all the wealth generated within a country; it excludes wealth brought in from outside.

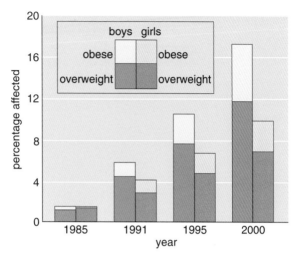

**Figure 1.24** Bar chart showing trends in the percentage of overweight and obese school children aged 7 to 18 years in large cities in China, 1985 to 2000. (Source: Wu, 2006, p. 363)

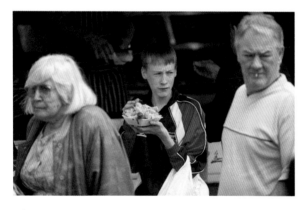

**Figure 1.25** Eating habits that led to obesity in older generations of a family can be passed on to younger members. (Photo: Mike Levers/Open University)

It has long been assumed that obesity occurs only among the most affluent individuals in developing countries like China. It appears, however, that as the wealth of a country increases, the obesity rate also rises but it predominates among people in *lower* socio-economic groups (Monteiro et al., 2004). Obesity also tends to 'run in families'.

◆ Can you suggest a reason, other than genetic inheritance, why overweight parents might have overweight children?

◆ Children are likely to copy the eating habits of their parents, not least because their parents purchase the family's food (Figure 1.25).

◆ In a number of countries, obesity rates are rising at a time when overall food consumption is declining. Can you suggest why?

◆ The amount of exercise that people take is very important in determining how fat they are. If exercise rates go down even faster than the decline in food consumption, then the rates of obesity will rise.

The determination of a person's body mass involves three processes: their energy intake, their energy use and the amount of energy stored in the body, mainly as fat. Briefly, energy derived from food is stored in a chemical form in our cells and is used in being active; chemical energy that is not used immediately is stored as fat. When humans were hunter-gatherers, and during the first agricultural revolution, energy-rich foods such as fatty meat and starchy cereals were not as plentiful as they are today. Being able to store surplus food as body fat in times of plenty was advantageous, because it enabled food shortages to be survived. But the tendency to 'put on weight' becomes a problem in the human zoo, where food is abundant and people are less active than when they worked on the land. The problem may be compounded by the fact that living in an environment where food is scarce caused our human ancestors to evolve a 'sweet tooth', that is, an ability to detect and prefer foods that are high in energy. An appetite for sweet foods and the ability to store excess energy have now become life-threatening.

## 1.6 Psychological problems in the human zoo

In 2004/5, the commissioners of health services for local communities in Britain (the Primary Care Trusts) spent over £7 billion (7000 million UK pounds) on mental health care. This represented 11% of their spending (Figure 1.26), more than on any other category of health care (King's Fund, 2006). Living in a developed urban society does not seem to make everyone happy. Worldwide, neuro-psychiatric conditions (that is, disorders of the brain linked with disorders

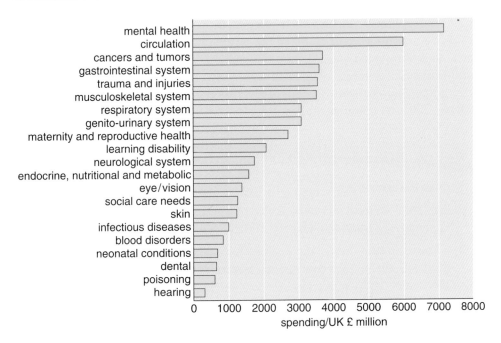

**Figure 1.26** Bar chart showing total spending in UK pounds sterling (£) on different categories of disease and disability by Primary Care Trusts in the UK in 2004/5. (Source: King's Fund, 2006, Figure 1, p. 2)

of the mind) account for 10.5% of the 'global burden of disease' (Murray and Lopez, 1997a), a measure of the impact of specific health conditions that takes account both of premature death and reduced quality of life. (You will learn about ways of measuring the disease burden in Chapter 2.)

Depression is one of the leading causes of poor health throughout the world and the WHO predicts that, by 2050, it will be second only to heart disease as the major preoccupation of doctors (WHO, 2007). Currently, neuro-psychiatric disorders make a much greater contribution to poor health in developed countries such as the UK than they do in sub-Saharan Africa and India, for example (Murray and Lopez, 1997a). While this suggests that mental health problems are more common in more affluent countries, such comparisons must be viewed with caution. The recognition and diagnosis of mental disorders varies much more from one country to another than is the case for 'physical' conditions such as heart disease or infections. In many developing countries, mental health problems are a growing cause for concern, for example among black South Africans.

## 1.6.1 Stress and its health effects

Urban life is widely regarded as being stressful, something that people try to get away from at the weekend and during holidays. Stress is an imprecise concept and psychologists have sought to define it more clearly (Carlson, 2001; Toates, 2007). It is important to differentiate between *stressors*, the external conditions that cause stress, and the way that people react to them. The **stress response** is defined as a physiological reaction occurring in the body, which is triggered by the perception of aversive or threatening situations.

In describing stress, a distinction is often made, as for many medical conditions, between acute and chronic forms of the condition. An **acute condition** is characterised by rapid onset, severe symptoms and short duration. A **chronic condition** lasts for a long time, involves slowly changing symptoms and often has a gradual onset. There are four main criteria for recognising chronic stress (Toates, 2007) as described in Box 1.6.

Hormones are chemical signalling molecules that circulate in the blood and trigger responses in specific tissues and organs in the body. Epinephrine is a hormone secreted by the suprarenal glands and was formerly known as *adrenalin*.

---

**Box 1.6** (Explanation) Features of chronic stress

1  Over time, a person is unable to remove or avoid one or more stressors.

2  The body secretes increased levels of a variety of hormones, such as epinephrine (eppy-neff-rin) and cortisol over a long period.

3  Chronic stress is associated with an increased probability of a range of illnesses, such as infections, heart attacks, high blood pressure, stomach ulcers and depression.

4  People under stress tend to engage in apparently pointless repetitive behaviour such as pacing up and down or nail-biting, or in extreme situations they may repeat self-harming acts such as pulling out chunks of hair or cutting their own skin.

◆  Can you recall another situation in which repetitive, stereotyped behaviour is quite common?

◆  Stereotypy occurs in many animals living in zoos (see Section 1.2.2), where they may be under prolonged stress, not least because they are held in confined spaces from which they cannot escape.

---

Of course what is experienced as stressful by one person might not have the same effect in another. Individual differences are enormous. Attempts within psychology to produce a water-tight definition have proven highly problematic and there is no precise consensus on what the term means. However, there is at least some agreement on the broad defining features. **Stress** seems invariably to convey the experience of being in an unpleasant situation, over a period of days, weeks or longer, in which you are unable to exert the control that you might have desired. The circumstances are not of your choosing, as in bereavement, divorce, excessive time pressure at work, or an unhappy marriage. You do not have the coping resources necessary to meet the demands of this unpleasant situation.

The stress response has its evolutionary origins in the 'fight or flight response'. Faced by a dangerous or aversive stimulus, such as a predator, an animal's nervous system responds immediately by triggering the secretion of epinephrine. This increases alertness and prepares the body for rapid movement. This response serves a person well in short-term emergencies, for example avoiding an oncoming bus, when the effects of the stress response are transitory. However, if you are stuck in a highly stressful job and subject to verbal bullying week after week, running away is not a viable solution. In such a situation, the body prepares itself for action by secreting the hormones that are normally triggered by

emergencies, but the 'fight or flight' response cannot be completed. Prolonged stressful situations that cannot easily be escaped can lead to harmful effects on health. For example, air-traffic controllers, especially those working at busy high-stress
airports, show an increased incidence of high blood pressure, relative to their counterparts in less stressful jobs (Figure 1.27).

◆ In Figure 1.27, what effect does age have on the difference in blood pressure between air traffic controllers in low- and high-stress airports?

◆ Blood pressure in the high-stress group is always above that in the low-stress group; but the gap widens after the age of about 40 years, when blood pressure rises sharply in both groups. This suggests that people may become less able to cope with prolonged stress as they get older.

Long-term exposure to stressful conditions can also affect the body's ability to cope with infections, leading to an increased incidence of ailments caused by common viruses and bacteria. People who suffer from 'cold sores', a condition caused by a virus, typically develop sores when they are tired or stressed. Post-traumatic stress disorder (PTSD) can also be induced by inescapable traumatic events, particularly those involving physical danger. The symptoms include recurrent bad dreams, intrusive memories of the traumatic event, impairment of social relationships and a profound feeling of helplessness (studies cited by Carlson, 2001).

For animals, including humans, that live in tightly knit social groups, social relationships can be a major source of stressful stimuli. For example, baboon colonies maintain a strict hierarchy in which more dominant individuals enjoy priority of access to food and other important resources. Knowing your place in the hierarchy can defuse stressful conflicts and allow more attention to focus on potential threats from outside the group. But in some parts of Africa, baboons have no natural predators and the biologist Robert M. Sapolsky observed that 'this leaves them hours each day to devote to generating social stress for each other' (quoted in Toates, 2007). This situation may be mirrored among young men (and in some countries such as the UK, also young women) in the towns and cities of our overcrowded world (Figure 1.28).

There is a widespread view that stress arises largely because modern urban living imposes an inappropriate 'work-life balance'. However, it is unlikely that stress in developed countries is due to people working too hard: all over the world, people now work less than they did in the past. In the UK in 1870, people worked an average of 2984 hours per year, or 57 hours per week; by 1998, the hours worked had fallen to 1489 hours, less than 30 hours per week (Maddison, 2001).

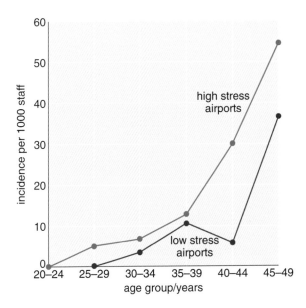

**Figure 1.27** Line graph showing the incidence rate (number of new cases per 1000 staff in a given period) of high blood pressure in different age-groups of air traffic controllers working at high-stress and low-stress airports. (Source: Carlson, 2001, Figure 18.6, p. 572)

PTSD is discussed further in another book in this series (Phillips, 2008).

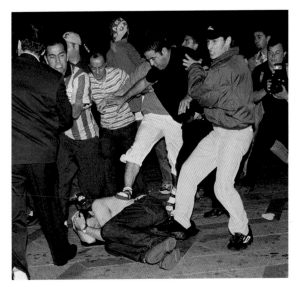

**Figure 1.28** Young men 'generating social stress for each other'. (Photo: Topham/TopFoto)

That working too hard is not a major cause of mental illness is supported by an analysis of the social and economic circumstances of people diagnosed with mental disorders (Meltzer et al., 2002). In people aged between 16 and 74 in the UK, being unemployed doubles the probability of having a mental disorder. Other factors associated with mental disorder are: low educational attainment, low income, being in debt, being single, divorced or separated, living in rented accommodation, and traumatic life events (e.g. divorce, death in the family, suffering an assault, being bullied at home).

Thus, in a developed country like the UK, mental illness, like most other health problems in countries all over the world, is most strongly associated with poverty and disadvantage. In the next chapter you will examine how data on disease and disability can be compared between richer and poorer nations, and consider what light this sheds on health in the human zoo.

## Summary of Chapter 1

1.1 Humans evolved as hunter-gatherers, living in small nomadic social groups. In the last 12 000 years, since settling in fixed agricultural communities, humans have come to live in a variety of artificial habitats, most notably large cities. More than half the world's population now lives in an urban environment.

1.2 Humans have had a major impact on planet Earth, destroying natural resources and causing pollution, particularly of the atmosphere and water sources. The impact on health has been exacerbated by rapid growth in the human population and by climate change.

1.3 Some features of present-day human anatomy and physiology are a legacy of evolutionary changes that were adaptive for our hunter-gatherer ancestors. The upright bipedal posture and compact pelvis make childbirth more difficult but enable us to run faster. The ability to store surplus food as body fat increases survival during food shortages, but increases the risk of obesity when food is plentiful and the need for exercise is low.

1.4 Countries are categorised according to a variety of criteria, including income and indicators of development such as access to education, health services, clean water and sanitation; the most commonly used categories are developed and developing countries. Combining data from large numbers of very diverse countries into a single group can disguise important differences between them.

1.5 The number of megacities containing more than 10 million inhabitants is rapidly increasing; the majority are in countries that cannot afford to provide adequate habitation, clean water and sanitation for a large proportion of their people.

1.6 Humans have become very mobile and travel further and more often than they did in the past. This facilitates the spread of infectious diseases.

1.7 The evolution and spread of antibiotic-resistant bacteria is accelerated by inappropriate use of antibiotics and is a growing problem worldwide.

1.8 Many measures of human health and well-being show clear differences between developed and developing countries, when data are presented in bar charts, scatter plots and line graphs.

1.9 People in developed countries enjoy a number of health advantages, such as greater life expectancy and lower infant mortality, but they incur a variety of health costs including greater rates of obesity and stress-related disorders.

## Learning outcomes for Chapter 1

After studying this chapter and its associated activities, you should be able to:

LO 1.1 Define and use in context, or recognise definitions and applications of, each of the terms printed in **bold** in the text. (Questions 1.1, 1.3, 1.5 and 1.6)

LO 1.2 Discuss the proposition that present-day human anatomy and physiology are a legacy of evolutionary changes that were adaptive for our hunter-gatherer ancestors, but which are not well suited to modern lifestyles in urban environments. (Question 1.1)

LO 1.3 Give examples of the impact that humans have had on natural environments on Earth. (Question 1.2)

LO 1.4 Describe the health problems that occur in megacities and other urban environments and as a result of the increased mobility of modern populations. (Question 1.3)

LO 1.5 Explain how countries are classified as 'developed' or 'developing' and give reasons for caution in interpreting data on the health experience of populations distinguished by this classification. (Question 1.4)

LO 1.6 Describe and interpret health data presented in tables, bar charts, scatter plots and line graphs. (Questions 1.5 and 1.6)

LO 1.7 Explain why failure to complete a course of antibiotics increases the risk that antibiotic-resistant bacteria will evolve and spread. (DVD Activity 1.1)

LO 1.8 Discuss the link between human diet, obesity and modern lifestyles and the consequences of obesity for human health. (Question 1.5)

LO 1.9 Describe the link between stress and modern lifestyles and give examples of stress-related illness. (Question 1.6)

If you are studying this book as part of an Open University course, you should also be able to:

LO 1.10 Access and search a database of newspaper articles on a particular topic, study two articles actively and make notes that enable you to compare and contrast them. (Questions in Activity C1 in the *Companion*)

## Self-assessment questions for Chapter 1

You had the opportunity to demonstrate LO 1.7 by answering questions in DVD Activity 1.1.

### Question 1.1 (LOs 1.1 and 1.2)

The chapter described the evolutionary 'trade-off' between the need to maximise running speed and the need to make childbirth reasonably safe for mothers and babies. What features of human anatomy and reproduction show evidence of this trade-off?

### Question 1.2 (LO 1.3)

Why are amphibians described as 'canaries in the coal mine' when it comes to the impact that humans are having on natural environments?

### Question 1.3 (LOs 1.1 and 1.4)

In 2003, an epidemic of an influenza-like illness called severe acute respiratory syndrome (SARS) began in Southern China and spread to Hong Kong, then to Toronto in Canada and Hanoi in Viet Nam. What does this example illustrate about the impact of modern lifestyles on the threat of infectious disease?

### Question 1.4 (LO 1.5)

In 2003, Singapore was classified as a high-income developed economy by the World Bank; its national income exceeded that of some Western European countries and New Zealand. The World Health Organization (WHO) classified it as a developing country. What reasons can you suggest for this discrepancy?

### Question 1.5 (LOs 1.1, 1.6 and 1.8)

Figure 1.29 shows the percentage of children in two age-groups in the USA who were classified as obese over a 40-year period. Describe the patterns in this bar chart and suggest a reason for the trend you observe.

### Question 1.6 (LOs 1.1, 1.6 and 1.9)

Why is it important to take account of the age of people in a study into the effects of stress on blood pressure?

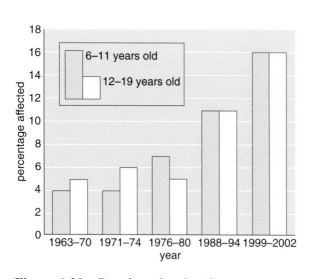

**Figure 1.29** Bar chart showing the percentage of children and teenagers in the USA classified as obese in a series of five surveys over a 40-year period. (Source: Nestle, 2006, p. 2529)

# CHAPTER 2

# MEASURING THE WORLD'S HEALTH

It's no longer a question of staying healthy. It's a question of finding a sickness you like.

(Jackie Mason, US comedian)

## 2.1 Epidemiology

In Chapter 1 we argued that many of the inhabitants of planet Earth are living in the equivalent of a 'human zoo' which is damaging health in ways that were unknown to our human ancestors. Evaluating how much 'health damage' is occurring, where and to whom, and whether it is getting better or worse over time, is the basis of **epidemiology** (epi-deemi-ol-ojee), the study of the occurrence, distribution, potential causes and control of diseases and disabilities in populations.

The development of strategies for addressing any aspect of human health begins with the gathering of statistics to determine the size of the problem and its distribution among the human population. Studying health data obtained from large populations can shed light on the possible underlying causes of ill health. For example, if a condition is more common in one age-group, or it affects males more than females, or is more often found in one country than in another, this may lead to **hypotheses** (clearly stated provisional and testable explanations) for the observed patterns, and then to targeted interventions to address the problem.

Two common measures used in epidemiology are worth clarifying from the outset. The **incidence** of a condition is the number of *new* cases diagnosed in a population in a given *period*, usually one year. The **prevalence** of a condition is the *total* number of people who have the condition at a particular *point in time*, regardless of how long they have been affected. Both the incidence and the prevalence are often expressed as a *rate*, i.e. the number of cases per 1000 people in the population in question (or per 10 000, or per 100 000 or per million, whichever is most convenient).

In Chapter 1, Figure 1.23 uses prevalence data to calculate the percentages shown and Figure 1.29 uses incidence data.

With these terms in mind, this chapter offers some insights into how health is measured and what can be learnt from routinely collected data about the state of human health at the start of the 21st century. It does not claim to be a comprehensive overview (this would take several books), but we aim to illuminate how profoundly the circumstances of people's lives affect their health, and to provide the foundations on which Chapter 3 builds.

## 2.2 Counting deaths

You may have noticed that all of the measures of 'health' presented so far in this book in fact relate to *deaths*, for example, life expectancy is based on an estimate of how many years will elapse between birth and death. Collecting **mortality data** (counts of deaths) is the commonest *indirect* way of measuring health (i.e. 'death' is being used as a proxy measure for 'absence of health').

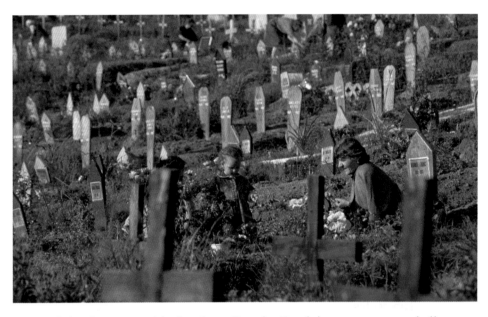

**Figure 2.1**   A graveyard in Sarajevo, Bosnia. Death is commemorated all over the world, and mortality data on age, gender, cause and date of death are among the most accessible statistics on which to base health reports. (Photo: Chris Sattiberger/Panos Pictures).

Deaths are more often recorded than episodes of illness, particularly in countries that lack a comprehensive system of data collection (Figure 2.1). Agencies such as the WHO publish a wealth of statistical reports on mortality from a wide range of causes, which are repeated at intervals so that changes can be tracked over time. Statistics on every cause of ill health are not collected every year and they are usually published at least two years (often much more) after the collection date, so it is difficult to present data all from the same year. In this chapter, we have selected the most recent statistics available at the time of writing, which means that in some tables and diagrams the data come from 2000 and in others from 2002.

### 2.2.1  Ranking deaths by cause

The 30 commonest causes of death worldwide in 1990 and 2002 are shown in Table 2.1, which enables you to see how their 'rank order' changed during this 12-year period. To avoid using a lot of noughts, deaths are given in millions as a decimal number.

If you are studying this book as part of an Open University course, go to Activity C2 in the *Companion* associated with this book now.

Diarrhoeal diseases, which are strongly associated with lack of access to clean drinking water and adequate sanitation (the focus of Chapter 3 of this book), appeared at number 4 in the ranking in Table 2.1 in 1990, but had fallen to seventh position by 2002 – a drop of 1.15 million deaths: (2.95 − 1.80 = 1.15 million or 1 150 000 fewer deaths from this cause).

◆   Look closely at Table 2.1. Which conditions moved above diarrhoeal diseases in 2002 compared with their ranking in 1990?

◆   The number of deaths from perinatal disorders/conditions (causing death within 7 days of birth) and chronic obstructive pulmonary disease (COPD)

COPD is the subject of another book in this series (Midgley, 2008).

**Table 2.1** The 30 commonest causes of death worldwide in 1990 compared with their ranking in 2002 (*conditions not in top 30 in 1990, **not in top 30 in 2002). (Source: data in columns 1 and 3: Murray and Lopez, 1997b, p. 1274; columns 4 and 5: WHO, 2004, Table 2, pp. 120–5)

| Rank in 1990 | Cause of deaths | No. of deaths (millions) in 1990 | No. of deaths (millions) in 2002 | Rank in 2002 |
|---|---|---|---|---|
| | *All causes combined* | 50.47 | 57.03 | |
| 1 | Ischaemic heart disease (due to blocked coronary arteries) | 6.26 | 7.21 | 1 |
| 2 | Cerebrovascular disease (e.g. strokes) | 4.38 | 5.51 | 2 |
| 3 | Lower respiratory tract infections (deep in the lungs) | 4.30 | 3.88 | 3 |
| 4 | Diarrhoeal diseases | 2.95 | 1.80 | 7 |
| 5 | Perinatal disorders/conditions (affecting babies in the first 7 days) | 2.44 | 2.46 | 6 |
| 6 | Chronic obstructive pulmonary disease (COPD, involves irreversible lung damage) | 2.21 | 2.75 | 5 |
| 7 | Tuberculosis (without HIV infection) | 1.96 | 1.57 | 8 |
| 8 | Measles | 1.06 | 0.61 | 20 |
| 9 | Road traffic accidents | 0.99 | 1.20 | 11 |
| 10 | Trachea, bronchus and lung cancers | 0.94 | 1.24 | 10 |
| 11 | Malaria | 0.86 | 1.27 | 9 |
| 12 | Self-inflicted injuries (including suicide) | 0.79 | 0.87 | 14 |
| 13 | Cirrhosis of the liver | 0.78 | 0.79 | 16 |
| 14 | Stomach cancer | 0.75 | 0.85 | 15 |
| 15 | Congenital abnormalities (birth defects) | 0.59 | 0.49 | 23 |
| 16 | Diabetes mellitus | 0.57 | 0.99 | 12 |
| 17 | Violence | 0.56 | 0.56 | 21 |
| 18 | Tetanus | 0.54 | 0.21 | ** |
| 19 | Nephritis/nephrosis (kidney disease) | 0.54 | 0.68 | 17 |
| 20 | Drowning | 0.50 | 0.38 | 29 |
| 21 | War injuries | 0.50 | 0.17 | ** |
| 22 | Liver cancer | 0.50 | 0.62 | 19 |
| 23 | Inflammatory heart diseases | 0.49 | 0.40 | 26 |
| 24 | Colon and rectum cancers | 0.47 | 0.62 | 18 |
| 25 | Protein-energy malnutrition | 0.37 | 0.26 | ** |
| 26 | Cancer of the oesophagus | 0.36 | 0.45 | 25 |
| 27 | Pertussis (whooping cough) | 0.35 | 0.29 | ** |
| 28 | Rheumatic heart disease | 0.34 | 0.33 | ** |
| 29 | Breast cancer | 0.32 | 0.48 | 24 |
| 30 | HIV/AIDS | 0.31 | 2.78 | 4 |
| * | Hypertensive heart disease (due to high blood pressure) | * | 0.91 | 13 |
| * | Maternal conditions (childbirth) | * | 0.51 | 22 |
| * | Alzheimer's disease and other dementias | * | 0.40 | 27 |
| * | Falls | * | 0.39 | 28 |
| * | Poisoning | * | 0.35 | 30 |

rose between 1990 and 2002, and they both overtook diarrhoeal diseases in the ranking, as the number of diarrhoea-related deaths decreased. The biggest movement anywhere in the table is the leap from 30th position in 1990 to 4th position in 2002 of deaths from HIV/AIDS.

When a condition causes rapidly accelerating numbers of deaths, it can shoot up the mortality ranking, pushing other conditions *down* the order even though their numbers are also *increasing* over time. This point is worth bearing in mind whenever you look at health data that has been rank ordered.

◆ Can you identify any conditions in Table 2.1 which ranked *lower* in 2002 than in 1990, even though the total number of deaths was *higher* in 2002?

◆ Perinatal disorders/conditions, road traffic accidents, self-inflicted injuries, cirrhosis of the liver and stomach cancer were all pushed lower in the ranking (despite increasing numbers of deaths) because deaths from some other conditions rose *even faster* and overtook them in the order.

In Figure 2.2, 'developed countries' combine all the 'developed' and the 'transitional economies' shown in Figure 1.10; the 'developing countries' in Figure 2.2 combine the 'developing' and the 'least developed' countries in Figure 1.10.

## 2.2.2 Proportional mortality and development status

The data in Table 2.1 summarise *what* people die of, but they do not reveal *which* people are at greater risk than others: young or old, male or female, rich or poor, for example. Nor do they reveal whether the *distribution* of global disease varies between different parts of the world. Data on the geographical distribution of mortality are presented in Figure 2.2a, which shows the number of deaths in millions in 2002 due to four main categories of cause. (These categories are distinguished in WHO databases (see Box 2.1); the WHO also publishes detailed data on all the individual causes *within* each category.) Figure 2.2b shows the same data converted into the *percentage* of the total number of global deaths contributed by each of the four categories. This way of representing deaths is known as the **proportional mortality** because it tells you what proportion (share) of all deaths occurs in each category.

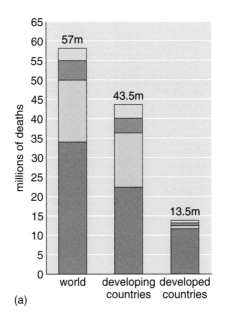

(a)

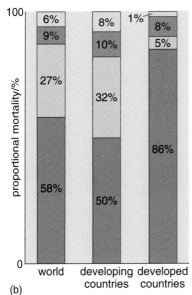

(b)

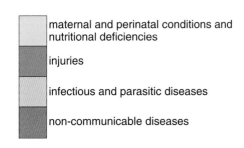

**Figure 2.2** Bar chart showing the main causes of mortality in 2002 for the world and for developed and developing countries. (a) Millions of deaths; (b) proportional mortality. The causal categories are described in the text. (Source: data derived from WHO, 2004)

**Box 2.1** (Explanation) Main categories of cause of death in WHO statistics

*Maternal and perinatal conditions and nutritional deficiencies* is a category distinguished by the WHO, which includes all deaths associated with childbirth or the first week of life, and deaths attributed directly to malnutrition.

The category termed **injuries** includes 'accidental deaths', e.g. in traffic accidents and falls, fires, drowning, poisoning and natural disasters, and 'non-accidental deaths' from self-inflicted injuries (principally suicide), violence, murder and warfare. Injuries resulting from traffic accidents are a growing global health problem (look back at Table 2.1).

The **infectious and parasitic diseases** are also known as 'communicable' diseases in WHO statistics because they can be passed on directly from one person to another, or indirectly via food, water, etc., or they are transmitted by intermediate organisms (e.g. mosquitoes transmit the malaria parasite). Most diseases in this category are caused by *microscopic agents* (i.e. visible only with the aid of a microscope, Figure 2.3), known collectively as **microbes** (or microorganisms), i.e. viruses, bacteria, fungal cells and single-celled parasites. (A parasite is an organism that lives on or in another organism, called its host, causing its host some degree of harm.) We referred to them as 'agents' not 'organisms' because viruses are not alive and they are not constructed from cells; you may also have heard of another type of infectious agent, the prions, which are unusual proteins. Some multicellular (composed of many cells) parasitic organisms, such as the tapeworms, live part of their lives inside the human body and are important causes of human disease. Many microbes and parasites are harmless to people, but those that cause disease are often referred to as **pathogens** ('pathogenic' means disease-causing), the term we use in this book.

**Non-communicable diseases** (so-called because they can't be transmitted from person to person) are mainly diseases that develop slowly over a long time period, and tend to affect people for a long time. They are often referred to as 'chronic' conditions. They include all forms of cancer, heart disease, respiratory diseases, diabetes, cirrhosis of the liver, and neuro-psychiatric conditions such as Alzheimer's disease and other dementias.

Traffic-related injuries are the subject of another book in this series, (Phillips, 2008).

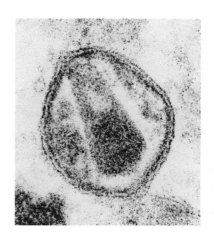

**Figure 2.3** The human immunodeficiency virus (HIV) is so small that it can only be photographed using a powerful electron microscope; this HIV 'particle' has been magnified 200 000 times. The thimble-shaped inner core contains the virus's genetic material and much of the outer layer is 'stolen' from the outer membrane of the human cell in which this virus was assembled. (Photo: Courtesy of the National Institute for Biological Standards and Control)

◆ What do the 'world' columns of Figure 2.2a and b reveal about the *relative importance* of deaths due to the four categories of main causes?

◆ Just over half (58%) of all deaths worldwide in 2002 were from chronic, non-communicable diseases (33.5 million), more than double the 15 million deaths (27% of the total) due to infectious and parasitic diseases. Injuries accounted for a further 5 million deaths (9% of the total), and maternal, perinatal and nutritional causes killed 3.5 million people (6% of the total).

◆ Figure 2.2a shows how the number of deaths was distributed between developed and developing countries. How would you sum up the differences?

◆ People in developing countries suffered 22 million deaths from chronic, non-communicable diseases, almost double the 11.5 million such deaths in developed countries. There were 20 times more deaths from infectious and parasitic diseases in developing countries (14 million) compared with developed countries (745 000), four times as many deaths from injuries and over 25 times as many deaths from maternal, perinatal and nutritional causes.

◆ Now look at Figure 2.2b. Which causal category contributes the largest percentage of deaths in developed countries, and how does this compare with the situation in developing countries?

◆ In both developed and developing countries, the largest percentage of deaths is due to *chronic, non-communicable* diseases: 86% of all deaths in developed countries and 50% of all deaths in developing countries.

People in richer nations tend to think of infectious and parasitic diseases as *the* major health problem in developing countries, so it may come as a surprise to note that *chronic* diseases are an even *bigger* problem. The WHO refers to developing countries as suffering the 'double jeopardy' of widespread infectious and parasitic diseases, coupled with rising rates of the chronic diseases familiar to the ageing populations of developed countries.

### 2.2.3 Scientific units and very large and very small numbers

The mention of infectious and parasitic diseases gives us an opportunity to make a short detour to show you how scientists and mathematicians communicate numerical information about, for example, how big a microbe is, how many cells there are in the human body, how far the Sun is from the Earth, or how much of a particular chemical there is in a given amount of water. To express such values accurately and unambiguously, two things are required: a standardised set of units and a way of dealing with very large and very small numbers.

**SI Units** (which stands for the French *Système Internationale*), is the term given to those units of measurement that scientists all over the world have agreed to use in their publications. For example, the *second* (abbreviated to s) is the standard unit for time, the *kilogram* (abbreviated to kg) is the standard unit for the mass of an object, and the *metre* (abbreviated to m) is the standard unit for the size of objects or the distance between objects. Metres are fine for describing objects and distances over a certain range, but become unwieldy when values are very large or very small. The units for describing objects and distances larger and smaller than one metre are shown in Table 2.2.

The third column in Table 2.2 shows how clumsy and long-winded communication would be if, for size and distance, the metre was the only unit available. The distance between Oxford and London is around 90 000 m; it is simpler to express this as 90 km. It is very much easier to say that the microbe that causes cholera is 1.3 μm (one point three micrometers) in length rather than 1.3 millionths of a metre. The same prefixes can be used with all other SI units (for example, kilograms, grams, milligrams, etc.).

**Table 2.2** SI units based on the metre (m). You will fill in the right-hand column later in this section.

| Name | Symbol | Value in metres (in words, fractions and as a decimal number) | Fill in the value as the power of ten |
|---|---|---|---|
| kilometre | km | one thousand metres (1000 m) | |
| metre | m | one metre (1 m) | |
| centimetre | cm | one hundredth of a metre (1/100 m or 0.01 m) | |
| millimetre | mm | one thousandth of a metre (1/1000 m or 0.001 m) | |
| micrometre | µm* | one millionth of a metre (1/1000 000 m or 0.000 001 m) | |
| nanometre | nm | one-thousand-millionth of a metre (1/1000 000 000 m or 0.000 000 001 m) | |
| picometre | pm | one-millon-millionth of a metre (1/1000 000 000 000 m or 0.000 000 000 001 m) | |

* The Greek letter µ (*mu,* pronounced 'meuw') and the prefix 'micro' both denote 'one-millionth' of a scientific unit such as the metre.

However, there still remains a problem when numerical values are *very* large or small. For example, the Earth is about 149 600 000 km from the sun. The method used for making such a number easier to express is called **powers of ten** notation (also known as *scientific* notation). Before we explain how this is used, look at Figure 2.4 (overleaf), which illustrates why this method is so useful. It shows the relative sizes of some of the pathogens that cause infectious and parasitic diseases, compared with the height of an average human adult and the length of the little finger of a newborn baby, so you have some idea of the scale. The diagram also gives the approximate number of cells in each of these examples. What may strike you about the numbers in Figure 2.4 is that the difference between the largest and the smallest is huge, and this makes it difficult to compare them 'at a glance'. Powers of ten notation enables you to do this.

For example, 100 is the same as $10 \times 10$ and this can be written as $10^2$ (ten 'squared'). The ten in $10^2$ is called the *base number* and the superscript 2 is called the *power*, so $10^2$ can also be said aloud as 'ten to the power two'. Of course there isn't any point in calling 100, 'ten to the power two' because it is an easily manageable number. However, the number of cells in a newborn baby's little finger contains a lot more noughts and converting it to a power of ten is helpful.

You met 'squared' numbers in Box 1.5 in the previous chapter, when we explained how body mass index (BMI) is calculated.

The baby's finger contains 1 billion cells, which is 1000 000 000, i.e. a 1 with 9 noughts after it. This is the same as $10 \times 10 \times 10 \times 10 \times 10 \times 10 \times 10 \times 10 \times 10$. Using powers of ten notation, 1 billion can be written as $10^9$ (the power is 9 because to get 1 billion, 10 has to be multiplied by itself a total of nine times) and spoken aloud as 'ten to the power nine' or just 'ten to the nine' for short.

◆ Express the number of cells in the adult human body as a power of ten. How would you say this number aloud?

◆ The number of cells is 1 million million, or 1000 000 000 000, i.e. a 1 with 12 noughts after it. This can be written as $10^{12}$ and spoken aloud as 'ten to the power twelve' or 'ten to the twelve' for short.

| | | number of cells | number as a power of ten | approximate length | visible with |
|---|---|---|---|---|---|
| 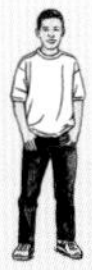 | adult human | 1000 000 000 000 (1 million million) | | 1.7 m | naked eye |
| 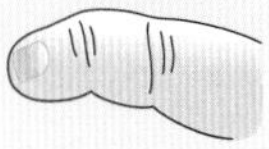 | newborn baby's little finger | 1000 000 000 (1 billion or 1000 million) | | 25 mm | |

| | | number of cells | length as a power of ten | approximate length | visible with |
|---|---|---|---|---|---|
| 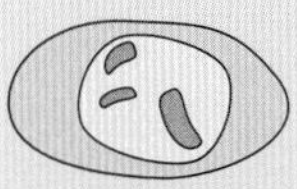 | malaria parasite (*Plasmodium*) | 1 | | 9 μm | |
| 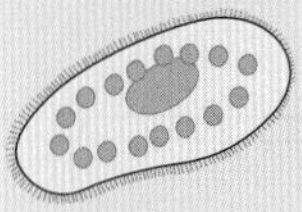 | parasite causing a diarrhoeal disease (*Cryptosporidium*) | 1 | | 5 μm | light microscope |
| 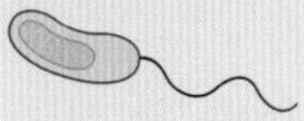 | bacterium causing cholera (*Vibrio cholerae*) | 1 | | 1.9 μm | |
| 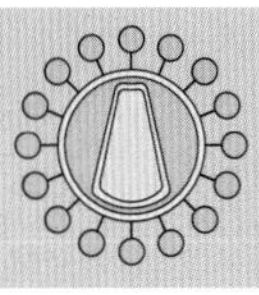 | human immunodeficiency virus (HIV) | 0 | | 0.1 μm | electron microscope |

**Figure 2.4** Comparative sizes (in metres) and numbers of cells in an adult human, the little finger of a newborn baby and some of the pathogens that cause infectious and parasitic diseases in humans. You will fill in the 'power of ten' column yourself. The numerical values are explained in the text and the sub-units of the metre are given in Table 2.2.

In Figure 2.4, in the space alongside '1 million million' (cells in an adult human), you can now write this huge number as $10^{12}$. Alongside '1 billion' (cells in a baby's finger) you can write $10^9$. The superscripts tell you that $10^{12}$ has been multiplied by 10 *three times more* than $10^9$; notice that when these numbers are written out in full, $10^{12}$ has *three more noughts* than $10^9$.

This is OK for expressing numbers larger than 10, but what about numbers smaller than 1? Small numbers can be described in powers of ten by *dividing* 1 by the power of ten. For example in Table 2.2, a millimetre is 1/1000th of a metre, or 1 *divided* by ten to the power three ($10^3$). To make this obvious it is written down as a *negative* power of 10 with a minus sign in front. So 1/1000th is written as $10^{-3}$.

◆ Table 2.2 states that a nanometre is one-thousand-millionth of a metre. Count the noughts in 1 nanometre and express this number as a negative power of ten.

◆ There are nine noughts in 1/1000 000 000, so a nanometre is $1/10^9$ m, or, using the negative powers of ten notation, 1 nanometre = $10^{-9}$ m (ten to the minus nine metres).

◆ Complete the right-hand column of Table 2.2 by filling in the powers of ten notation for the other sub-units of 1 metre.

◆  1 centimetre = $10^{-2}$ m (ten to the minus two metres), 1 millimetre = $10^{-3}$ m, 1 micrometre = $10^{-6}$ m, and 1 picometre = $10^{-12}$ m.

In Figure 2.4, the length of the malaria parasite *Plasmodium* is given as 9 μm (9 micrometres). In powers of ten notation this would be written as $9 \times 10^{-6}$ m (nine times ten to the minus six metres), i.e. this single-celled organism is nine one-millionths of a metre in length. Write $9 \times 10^{-6}$ m into the 'powers of ten' column in Figure 2.4 in the row for malaria.

◆  Convert the lengths in mm of *Cryptosporidium* and *Vibrio cholerae* into the equivalent lengths in metres, using powers of ten notation.

◆  The lengths are $5 \times 10^{-6}$ m and $1.9 \times 10^{-6}$ m, respectively. (Write these values into Figure 2.4.)

The length of an HIV particle is given in micrometres in Figure 2.4 as 0.1 μm. This is the same as $0.1 \times 10^{-6}$ m, but it isn't written like this in scientific notation. There is a convention that if a power of ten is multiplied by another number, the multiplier should always be between 1 and 10. If the size of the HIV particle is written as $0.1 \times 10^{-6}$ m, the multiplier is 0.1, which breaks the convention. So how can we change the multiplier to a number between 1 and 10 and still express the size of the virus correctly?

This is how it's done. We can increase 0.1 to 1 by *multiplying* it by 10:

$0.1 \times 10 = 1.$

The value of the multiplier now fits the convention (it's between 1 and 10), but we have to counterbalance this increase by *dividing* the power by 10.

$10^{-6} \div 10 = 10^{-7}.$

$0.1 \times 10^{-6}$ is the *same* as $1 \times 10^{-7}$, but the preferred version in scientific notation is $1 \times 10^{-7}$. Write the length of an HIV particle in the 'power of ten' column of Figure 2.4 as $1 \times 10^{-7}$ m.

Figure 2.4 showed a range of dimensions that represent typical sizes in the 'biological world'; other branches of science (e.g. astronomy) cover much larger distances and some (e.g. atomic physics) use much smaller distances. You will often encounter powers of ten notation in scientific writing involving very large or very small numbers, and there are some examples in Chapter 3. However, you should note one exception: epidemiologists *rarely* use powers of ten when they express the very large numbers common in health statistics; for example, '1 million deaths' from a particular condition is not usually written as $10^6$ deaths. This takes us back to the measurement of mortality.

### 2.2.4  Mortality rates in different countries

A great deal of information can be extracted from the 'raw counts' of how many people died in a given year, but this type of data cannot be used to make direct comparisons of the health status of different countries.

◈ Suppose you compared the total number of deaths from a particular cause (e.g. respiratory diseases) in China and in the United Kingdom (UK) in the same year. Why would this comparison be unable to tell you which country had the worst respiratory health problem?

◆ The population size varies so enormously between these two countries and this has to be taken into account (e.g. China has around 2 billion people, whereas the UK has around 60 million). China is certain to have a larger *number* of deaths from respiratory diseases than the UK in any year, simply because it has a larger population. The 'raw counts' would be unable to tell you whether the smaller number of UK deaths represented a worse or better health record than in China.

Comparisons of mortality data between different countries, or different groups within a population (e.g. everyone over or under a certain age; males and females, etc.) can only be made if the number of deaths *and* the number of people in the affected population are combined to calculate a **mortality rate**. You have already met two examples in Chapter 1, the *infant mortality rate* (IMR, see Figure 1.20) and the *child mortality rate* (Table 1.1). These are proxy measures for the health of babies in their first 12 months and children under 5 years of age respectively, and both are expressed as the number of deaths for every 1000 babies born alive.

*Screening for Breast Cancer* (Parvin, 2007) is the subject of another book in this series.

Many other forms of mortality rate can be calculated, including for other age groups and for women and men separately. For example, the mortality rate for breast cancer, which is rare among men, is expressed as the number of deaths from breast cancer relative to the number of *women* in the population.

◈ What effect would it have if breast cancer mortality were expressed as the number of deaths relative to the total number of *people* in a population?

◆ The overall mortality rate would be about *half* the actual rate in women, because about half the population are men; including them in calculating the mortality rate for a condition that very few men develop would have a 'diluting' effect on the rate. (Women are the population most *at risk* of developing breast cancer.)

## 2.3 Estimating the burden of ill health

Data on mortality provide no information about the extent of long-term disease or disability in a population, or its effects on the quality of individual lives. The technical term for disease and disability is morbidity, and the **morbidity rate** is the number of cases of a disorder in a population, relative to the total number of people *at risk* of developing it. Like mortality rates, morbidity rates are expressed as the number of cases per 1000 or per 10 000, or whatever is the most convenient denomination, right up to cases per million population. And again, like mortality rates, the population on which the rate is based generally excludes people who could not develop the condition, so the morbidity rate is expressed for those who *are* at risk. Counting the number of cases of a disorder is notoriously difficult, however.

◆ Can you suggest some reasons why? (Think back to the definitions of incidence and prevalence at the start of this chapter.)

◆ You may have noted that decisions about *what* to count aren't straightforward and there are bound to be many uncertainties in the data. If you try to count all the *new* cases diagnosed in a year (the incidence), can you be sure that the diagnoses are accurate? If you try to count the prevalence (all cases present at one point in time), have you found them all? Illnesses are often self-treated, so they go unrecorded, or people conceal them, or the data-collection system is inadequate or it fails to reach remote populations. Some conditions have periods of remission, or they fluctuate unpredictably (e.g. asthma, multiple sclerosis), so do you leave out all the people who are not showing symptoms in the data-collection period? Extracting 'case counts' from medical records may also be tricky; the same individual may consult a health professional many times during the same illness.

### 2.3.1 Disability adjusted life years

In an attempt to improve the consistency of morbidity data, the WHO and the World Bank began the *Global Burden of Disease* (GBD) project in 1992, to provide numerical estimates of all significant causes of death, illness and disability for each of the 192 member states of the WHO. Data are also collected on a variety of important variables that may influence health, such as geography, age-group, gender, socio-economic circumstances, national wealth, the amount spent on health services, the number of health workers, and many other factors.

As well as mortality rates, the GBD project publishes morbidity data using an internationally recognised measure called the **disability adjusted life year** (or **DALY** – pronounced 'daily'), which aims to reflect the real impact of each disease, disorder or disability on people's lives (Figure 2.5). The calculation is complex, but in essence DALYs combine an estimate of the number of years lived with a reduced quality of life, taking into account the severity of the

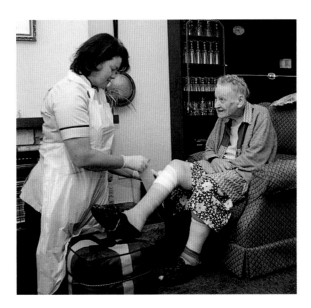

**Figure 2.5**   The extent to which disability adversely affects a person's life is estimated in disability adjusted life years (DALYs), taking into account the severity of the condition, the age of the person and whether it causes premature death. (Photo: Mike Levers/ Open University)

condition (every condition is assigned a 'weighting factor' to reflect this), *and* the number of years of life lost if the person dies prematurely, based on their age and the average life expectancy in that population.

If the total number of disability adjusted life years suffered by all the people affected by a condition in a particular country, in a given year, are added together, some very large numbers result. For example, a total of 587 000 DALYs were due to depression in the population of the UK in 2002; that's 587 000 years of life that would have been lived in good health, if there was no depression. Read in isolation, such a figure is not very informative; does it mean that people in the UK are very depressed, or not? Estimates of DALYs become most useful when they are compared with one another.

*Comparing morbidity between countries*

Table 2.3 compares the total DALYs for a small number of conditions in the UK and in the United Republic of Tanzania (URT). The comparison between the disease burden in one of the world's richest countries and in one of the poorest is revealing.

Table 2.3 shows that people in Tanzania suffered nearly three times as many DALYs in total as people in the UK in 2002, despite the fact that its population is much smaller. This makes the point that not just mortality, but also morbidity, is generally worse in developing than in developed countries.

◆ Table 2.3 shows that more than twice as many DALYs were due to depression in the UK than in Tanzania. Does this mean that people in Tanzania (on average) suffer *less* from depression than people in the UK? (Hint: look at the size of each population.)

The UK and the URT are next to each other in alphabetical listings of countries in WHO statistical tables. This proximity makes it very easy to compare their health and development indicators.

**Table 2.3** Estimated total number of disability adjusted life years (DALYs) in 2002 due to all causes combined and due to selected conditions in the United Republic of Tanzania (URT) and the United Kingdom (UK). (Data derived from WHO, 2003, Statistical Annex, Table 3)

| Condition | DALYs | |
| --- | --- | --- |
| | Tanzania (URT) | UK |
| *DALYs due to all causes* | 20.24 million | 7.56 million |
| DALYs due to: | | |
|     diarrhoeal diseases | 1.06 million | 18 000 |
|     depression | 231 000 | 587 000 |
|     road traffic accidents | 374 000 | 110 000 |
|     alcohol | 62 000 | 278 000 |
|     breast cancer | 12 000 | 154 000 |
|     chronic obstructive pulmonary disease (COPD) | 49 000 | 367 000 |
| *Total population number* | 36.28 million | 59.07 million |

◆ In one sense it does. Even though the total population of the UK is larger than that of Tanzania, it isn't *twice* as large, so the fact that the UK has a much larger number of DALYs due to depression cannot be accounted for simply by having a bigger population. But you may have wondered if all cases of depression were being diagnosed in Tanzania; uncertainty about diagnostic accuracy and about data collection could mean that the true number is a lot bigger.

Another way of evaluating the relative impact of depression in the two countries is to calculate the *percentage* of all DALYs that are due to depression. You can do this from the data in Table 2.3. For example, the percentage in the UK is calculated by dividing the number of DALYs due to depression (587 000) by the total number of DALYs due to all causes (7.56 million = 7 560 000); the result is multiplied by 100 to express it as a percentage. This is the **proportional morbidity**, the 'share' of all DALYs that are due to depression.

$$\frac{587\,000}{7\,560\,000} \times 100 = 7.8\%$$

◈ Use a calculator (if you have one) to work out the percentage of all DALYs that are due to depression in Tanzania. (20.24 million = 20 240 000)

◆ $$\frac{231\,000}{20\,240\,000} \times 100 = 1\%$$

This confirms that depression accounts for a smaller proportion of DALYs in Tanzania than it does in the UK.

◈ In Table 2.3, which condition showed the biggest difference between these countries?

◆ Diarrhoeal diseases, which accounted for 60 times more DALYs in Tanzania than in the UK. (If you worked out the percentage of all DALYs due to these diseases, they contributed 5% of all DALYs in Tanzania in 2002, compared with 0.2% in the UK, a 25-fold difference.)

Once a reliable method for gathering morbidity data has been developed, disease statistics can be collected at regular intervals to determine if there are any significant trends. Policy-makers can tell, for example, if a particular disease or cause of disability is becoming more common over time, and whether efforts to combat it are having any effect.

### 2.3.2 Evaluating the impact of disease risk factors

A powerful way of using morbidity data to shed light on the causes of disease is to calculate how much of the global burden of disease can be attributed to different **risk factors**. A disease risk factor is anything which is *associated* in a population with an increased chance of developing a particular disease; that is, when the incidence of the disease is examined in different populations it is found to occur more frequently in those who have been exposed to the risk factor than in those who have not, or whose exposure level has been lower.

However, you cannot assume a *causal connection* just because two variables are *associated*. For example, smoking tobacco is strongly associated with lung cancer; the disease is rare in lifelong non-smokers and common in people who smoke. But this statistic on its own cannot prove that smoking *causes* lung cancer; the conclusive proof that it *does* came from laboratory experiments. The statistical association between lung cancer and smoking is what alerted health scientists to investigate whether there was a causal connection.

### The top ten global disease risk factors

Bear this in mind as you look at Table 2.4, which presents data on deaths and DALYs for the ten most significant global disease risk factors in 2000. Some of these are medical symptoms of poor health (e.g. underweight, high blood pressure), some are aspects of human behaviour (e.g. unsafe sex, alcohol consumption) and some are environmental factors (e.g. unsafe water and/or poor sanitation, smoke from indoor cooking fires). These are ranked according to their percentage contribution to global estimates of DALYs.

◆ If Table 2.4 were to be reorganised to rank the ten risk factors in order of the number of *deaths*, how would the result compare with the ranking based on DALYs? (To put it another way, would a ranking based on *mortality* be similar to or different from a ranking based on *morbidity*?)

◆ Underweight comes out top in DALYs (it contributed 9.5% of all the years of life lost to all disabling conditions globally in 2000), but it contributes less to *mortality* than three other risk factors: high blood pressure (over 7 million deaths), tobacco consumption (almost 5 million deaths) and high cholesterol (4.4 million deaths). So it ranks fourth as a cause of death.

This reflects the fact that DALYs incorporate measures of *both* mortality *and* morbidity: underweight scores so highly as a proportion of the global burden

**Table 2.4** DALYs associated with the top ten worldwide disease risk factors in 2000, ranked in order of their percentage contribution to the global burden of disease (GBD), with the total number of deaths attributable to each risk factor (in millions). (Source: Rodgers et al., 2004, Table 1, p. 46)

| Type of health risk | Specific risk factors | DALYs as a % of GBD (rank) | Deaths (millions) |
|---|---|---|---|
| childhood and maternal under-nutrition | underweight | 9.5 (1st) | 3.75 |
| sexual and reproductive health | unsafe sex | 6.3 (2nd) | 2.88 |
| overweight/physical inactivity | high blood pressure | 4.4 (3rd) | 7.14 |
| addictive substances | tobacco | 4.1 (4th) | 4.91 |
| addictive substances | alcohol | 4.0 (5th) | 1.80 |
| unsafe water/poor sanitation | deficient water supply and sanitation | 3.7 (6th) | 1.73 |
| nutrition/physical inactivity | high cholesterol | 2.8 (7th) | 4.42 |
| indoor smoke from solid fuels | indoor cooking fires | 2.6 (8th) | 1.62 |
| childhood and maternal under-nutrition | iron deficiency anaemia | 2.4 (9th) | 0.84 |
| nutrition/physical inactivity | obesity: high body mass index (BMI) | 2.3 (10th) | 2.59 |

of disease because it contributes to the deaths of large numbers (most of them children aged under five), and it also makes a lot of people ill and reduces their quality of life over very long periods.

*Risk factors can vary with gender and age*

Global, regional or national health statistics can be analysed in other ways, for example by gender, or by age. Figure 2.6 presents global data on mortality and morbidity for five major disease risk factors, chosen to illustrate their different impacts on males and females. Each of the small bar charts shows how the total mortality and the total morbidity (in DALYs) associated with each risk factor is 'shared' between males and females. For example, bar chart (a) shows that 55% of all deaths attributed to obesity occur in females, who also suffer 53% of all DALYs due to its disabling effects.

◆ Which of the risk factors in Figure 2.6 show the greatest difference in mortality and morbidity between males and females worldwide?

◆ Males are much more likely to sustain occupational injuries and they are at substantially greater risk of death and disease than females from the damaging effects of alcohol and tobacco.

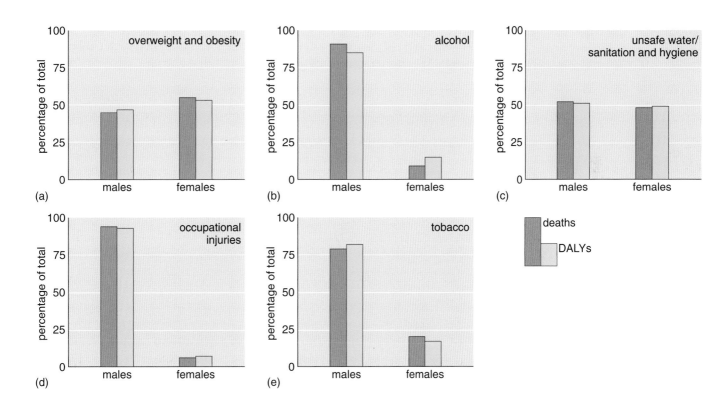

**Figure 2.6** Bar charts showing the relative impact of five disease risk factors on global health in males and females in 2000: charts (a) to (e) show what percentage of the total mortality and the total DALYs associated with each risk factor is experienced by males and by females. (Data derived from Rodgers et al., 2004, Table 3, p. 50)

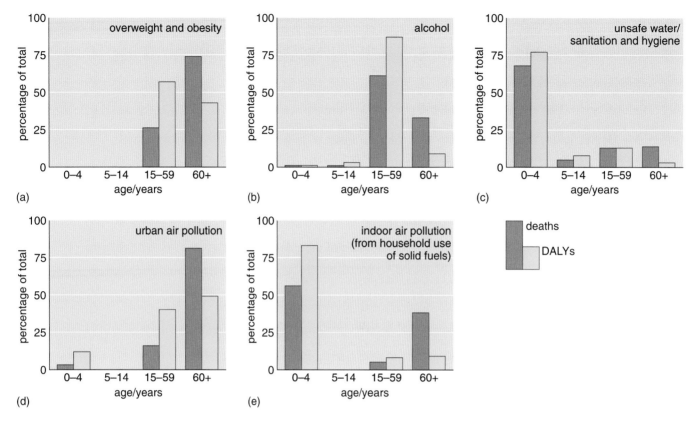

**Figure 2.7** Bar charts showing the relative impact of five disease risk factors on global health in different age-groups in 2000: charts (a) to (e) show what percentage of the total mortality and the total DALYs associated with each risk factor is experienced in each age-group. (Source: as Figure 2.6)

Figure 2.7 presents data on five disease risk factors (three of them are the same as in Figure 2.6), chosen to illustrate their effects on different age-groups.

◆ Which of the risk factors in Figure 2.7 have the greatest impact on health among children aged 0–4 years?

◆ Unsafe water, poor sanitation and hygiene, and indoor air pollution from household use of solid fuels.

Indoor smoke pollution and its effects on respiratory health are explored in another book in this series (Midgley, 2008).

These risks are very high on a global scale because of the huge number of children in developing countries who drink and wash in water contaminated by human and animal sewage, and who are routinely exposed to smoke from indoor cooking stoves, which predisposes them to respiratory diseases. Notice in Figure 2.7e that indoor smoke also disproportionately affects people over the age of 60 years, who have been exposed to it for most of their lives.

In the next chapter of this book, we focus on the first of these risk factors, access to clean water and adequate sanitation, as we examine the properties of water that make it essential to life on planet Earth.

## Summary of Chapter 2

2.1 Population health can be measured by counting deaths (mortality data) due to specific causes, and by counting cases of disease, disorder and disability (morbidity data).

2.2 Comparisons of mortality and morbidity data between regions, countries or groups within a population are best expressed either as a *rate*, taking into account the number in the relevant population, or as a *proportion* or *percentage* of the total number of deaths or cases of disease.

2.3 The rapid rise in HIV/AIDS over the past 20 years has pushed several other important health conditions down the global ranking of causes of death or disease, even though their numbers are still rising.

2.4 The disability adjusted life year (DALY) is a measure of the total number of years lived with a disease, disorder or disability, taking its severity into account, and the years lost due to premature death.

2.5 Chronic non-communicable diseases cause the largest proportion of deaths and DALYs in both developed and developing countries, but the latter also suffer the 'double jeopardy' of much higher rates of infectious and parasitic diseases, injuries, maternal and perinatal conditions and nutritional deficiencies.

2.6 Very large or very small numbers can be expressed in scientific writing (but not usually in health statistics) using powers of ten notation.

2.7 The burden of disease due to a specific condition can be associated with specific disease risk factors, but a statistical association does not (on its own) prove that the risk factor *causes* the disease.

2.8 The relative importance of specific causes of mortality and morbidity can vary significantly between developed and developing countries, and between different age-groups and genders.

## Learning outcomes for Chapter 2

After studying this chapter and its associated activities, you should be able to:

LO 2.1 Define and use in context, or recognise definitions and applications of, each of the terms printed in **bold** in the text. (Questions 2.2 and 2.3)

LO 2.2 Summarise, interpret and comment on morbidity and mortality data presented in diagrams and tables like those in this chapter. (Questions 2.1, 2.2 and 2.3)

LO 2.3 Recognise and give examples to illustrate what is meant by the 'double jeopardy' of the burden of infectious and parasitic diseases and chronic non-communicable diseases in developing countries. (Question 2.4)

LO 2.4 Express very large and very small numbers using powers of ten notation, and assign the correct units to measurements of length in metres. (Question 2.5)

LO 2.5 Identify some of the top ten global disease risk factors and the disease conditions with which they are associated; give examples of disease risk factors that illustrate a greater association with disease in males or females, or with people in different age-groups. (Question 2.3)

If you are studying this book as part of an Open University course, you should also be able to:

LO 2.6 Express large numbers as their decimal equivalents in units of millions or thousands. (Questions in Activity C2 in the *Companion*)

## Self-assessment questions for Chapter 2

### Question 2.1 (LO 2.2)

Look back at Table 2.1. Which condition had fallen the furthest down the ranking in 2002, compared with its position in 1990?

### Question 2.2 (LOs 2.1 and 2.2)

Calculate the proportional morbidity (in DALYs) from road traffic accidents in Tanzania and the UK in 2002, from the data given in Table 2.3. Express your answer to one decimal place (i.e. you need only give the first number after the decimal point; calculators will give the answer to several decimal places.)

### Question 2.3 (LOs 2.1 and 2.5)

Which of the disease risk factors referred to in Figure 2.7 has the largest impact on the disease burden in people aged 15–59 years?

### Question 2.4 (LOs 2.1, 2.3 and 2.5)

(a) Give examples of some important risk factors associated with the high rates of infectious and parasitic diseases in developing countries.

(b) Which risk factors are associated with the even higher rates of chronic non-communicable diseases in developing countries?

(c) Which of the risk factors you identified in (a) and (b) are *not* significant causes of disease in developed countries?

### Question 2.5 (LO 2.1 and 2.4)

The length of the bacterium *Mycobacterium tuberculosis* (which causes TB) is 0.3 μm. Express this number in metres, using powers of ten notation.

# CHAPTER 3

# WATER AND HUMAN HEALTH

We shall not finally defeat AIDS, tuberculosis, malaria, or any of the other infectious diseases that plague the developing world until we have also won the battle for safe drinking-water, sanitation and basic health care.

(Kofi Annan, United Nations Secretary-General (2005)
*The International Decade for Action* 2003–2015)

## 3.1  Water as a global resource

Freshwater is a natural resource that is vital for human survival and health. The Earth is a very wet planet, but only 2.53% of its water is fresh; the rest is seawater (UNESCO, 2003). There is currently much concern about the capacity of the Earth's freshwater resources to sustain human life and health in the near future. One estimate suggests that, if current trends continue, by 2050, when the global human population will reach almost nine billion people, seven billion people in 60 countries will be short of water unless action is taken (UNESCO, 2003). Half the human population will be short of water by 2025.

◆ Can you suggest some reasons why such dire predictions are being made?

◆ They arise because people are using water at an increasing rate, the human population is expanding, and predicted patterns of climate change are expected to reduce water availability in many parts of the world, while increasing it in others.

As well as being concerned about the *quantity* of water available for humans, governments and international agencies are much concerned with its *quality*. Naturally occurring water is never pure, but contains a wide variety of dissolved substances, some of which are harmful to health, as well as microbes, some of which are pathogens, i.e. they can cause illness. You will return to health issues related to the pollution of water, by chemicals and by microbes, in Sections 3.4 to 3.6.

If predictions about a shortage of water for half the human population in 2025 seem alarming but far away, it is important to point out that, for many people, a water crisis is already a daily experience. As you will see later, many people in the world already face the severe adverse consequences for their health of having insufficient water and water that is also polluted. This is particularly true in Africa (Figure 3.1, overleaf).

A global water crisis is already apparent to those who look beyond humans and consider what is happening to other species. Planet Earth is at the beginning of a mass extinction event that is eliminating species at a faster rate than at any time in the history of the planet. This is the sixth mass extinction event in Earth's history; the fifth saw the extinction of the dinosaurs, around 70 million years ago. While much media attention is focused on the destruction of tropical forests around the world, it is in fact biodiversity in the world's freshwater habitats that is declining the fastest; you will return to this in Section 3.6.

1 billion = 1000 million

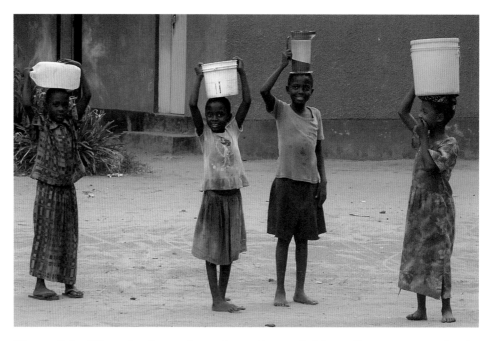

**Figure 3.1**   Water for domestic use has to be carried long distances every day in many parts of Africa, mainly by women and girls. (Source: Global Environment Teaching, East Africa)

Planet Earth contains an enormous amount of water, but only a tiny fraction of it is available, as freshwater, to plants and animals, including humans that live on land. As Figure 3.2 shows, only about 0.01% of the world's total freshwater is readily available to terrestrial life.

Here are some more facts about the world's freshwater resources to bear in mind as you study this chapter (Lannoo et al., 2006):

- Freshwater is unevenly distributed throughout the world, e.g. Canada has 30 times as much freshwater available to each of its citizens as China.

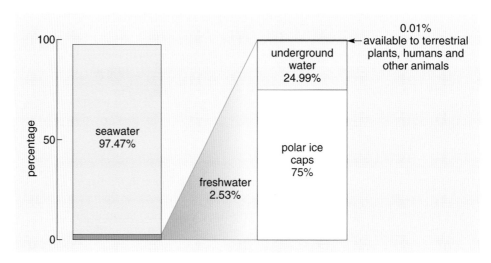

**Figure 3.2**   The distribution of the world's water resources. (Source: based on data quoted in Lannoo et al., 2006)

- Freshwater is being contaminated by saltwater influxes (tidal waves, rising sea levels), human waste and other by-products of human activity (e.g. industrial chemicals, acid rain), as well as agricultural fertilisers, pesticides and herbicides.

- Since 1950, the number of people on Earth has increased from 2.5 to 6.5 billion, and the per capita use of freshwater (i.e. the amount each person uses annually) has tripled. By 2050 the human population is predicted to reach 8.9 billion; per capita water use is also expected to continue to increase.

- More than 60% of all freshwater used in the world is diverted for agriculture.

## 3.2 The global water cycle

The flow of water through the land, the atmosphere and the sea is shown in Figure 3.3.

The route by which most water enters the atmosphere is evaporation from the sea. Much smaller amounts of water enter the atmosphere from the land and from rivers and lakes.

Water vapour in the atmosphere condenses into clouds and falls as precipitation (rain, hail or snow). The distribution of rainfall across the planet is very uneven, with some regions receiving rain all year round, and some receiving none at all

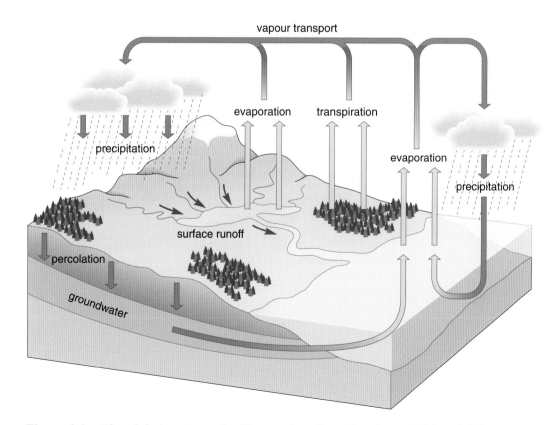

**Figure 3.3** The global water cycle. (Source: based on Houghton, 2004, p. 155)

(Figure 3.4). Some of the water that falls on the land runs into streams and thence into lakes, rivers and the sea; some of it evaporates back into the atmosphere and a lot of it percolates deep into the ground, where it becomes groundwater. Groundwater, extracted by means of wells, is an important source of water for people, especially in those parts of the world where rainwater is insufficient to meet their needs. Percolation through the ground purifies water by filtration so that water that emerges from the ground at natural springs is typically very free of microbes.

**Transpiration** is the release of water vapour by plants (Figure 3.3). Plants take in carbon dioxide from the atmosphere, and release oxygen. To maintain a flow of nutrients through their stems and leaves they take up water in their roots and release it as water vapour through tiny holes in their leaves, called stomata, through which they also take in carbon dioxide. A recent study suggests that, because carbon dioxide levels in the atmosphere are rising through the burning of fossil fuels, plants don't need to keep their stomata as wide open as they used to in order to obtain the carbon dioxide they need. As a consequence plants are now releasing less water into the atmosphere than they did in the past (Gedney et al., 2006; Matthews, 2006). This represents a very subtle consequence of climate change that affects the global water cycle, and makes the important point that the global ecosystem is very complex, and that a change in one component can have wide-ranging and unexpected consequences.

An important component of the water cycle, not shown in Figure 3.3, is human intervention in the form of sanitation systems. Water-borne human waste is collected in sewers, treated in sewage plants and returned, as cleaner water, to the

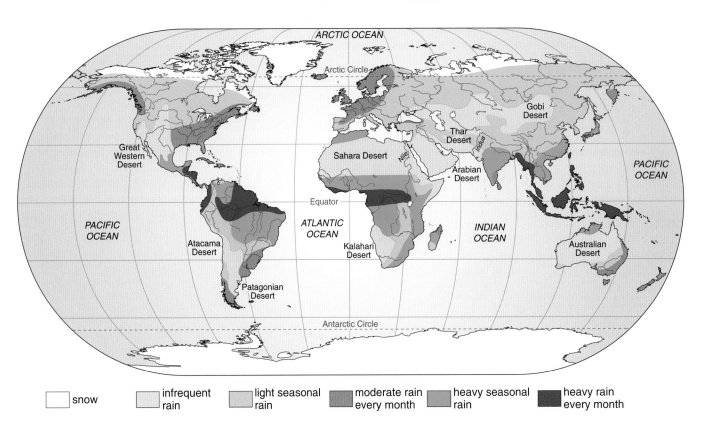

**Figure 3.4**   Map showing world rainfall.

water cycle, into rivers or the sea. The primary function of sewage treatment is to break down faeces and remove harmful microbes from the water. Sewage plants also have a role to play in removing harmful chemicals from water. In heavily populated parts of the world, water passing through sanitation systems represents a substantial proportion of the water flow in rivers. The River Lea, which runs from Hertfordshire in England into the River Thames, would probably cease to flow for much of the year were it not for the output from sewage plants (Brown, 2002).

The population in many of the world's megacities (Section 1.2.6) is growing so fast that the development of effective sewage systems is not keeping pace. In cities such as Karachi, in Pakistan, the water supply, mostly from groundwater, is heavily polluted by untreated sewage and contains high levels of bacteria (Rahman et al., 1997).

## 3.3 The distribution of water and its use by people

People in many parts of the world currently face a chronic shortage of water; this is a developing crisis that is expected to get worse. As you read in Section 3.1, several factors underlie this dire prediction. In addition, climate change is expected to cause major changes in the distribution of freshwater. The uneven distribution of freshwater across the world is illustrated in Table 3.1.

◆ From the data in Table 3.1, which continent is facing the greatest water crisis?

◆ Asia. It contains nearly two thirds of the world's human population, but only one third of its available freshwater.

◆ Compare the data in Table 3.1 with the world rainfall map in Figure 3.4. Is water availability in different regions reflected in the pattern of rainfall?

◆ Generally, yes, it is. The regions of highest water availability (Asia, South America) have high rainfall. The region with the lowest water availability (Australia) has low rainfall.

**Table 3.1** Distribution of the world's human population and available fresh water across six continents. (Source: data derived from UNESCO, 2003, Figure 1, p. 9)

| Continent | Proportion of world's human population/% | Proportion of world's available freshwater/% |
|---|---|---|
| North and Central America | 8 | 15 |
| South America | 6 | 26 |
| Europe | 13 | 8 |
| Africa | 13 | 11 |
| Asia | 60 | 36 |
| Australia and Oceania | 1 | 5 |

◆ Which region does not fit this pattern?

◆ Africa has high rainfall (Figure 3.4), but rather low water availability (Table 3.1).

The reason for this is that rainfall in Africa is concentrated near the Equator, but is low in southern Africa, where many people live.

People use water for a variety of purposes. As well as water for drinking, people use water to wash in, for sanitation, to irrigate the land for crops, to give to livestock, as a source of food (fishing), for transport and for recreation. The major categories of water use, on a global scale, are summarised in Figure 3.5, which shows that water use increased up to 1995 and how it is predicted to continue to increase up to 2025.

◆ What is the most significant use of water worldwide?

◆ Agriculture: in 2025 it will account for 60% of all the water extracted from natural water resources (just over 3000 km$^3$ in the total of just over 5000 km$^3$).

◆ Which of the factors discussed in Section 3.1 account for the fact that water extraction is increasing?

◆ Increasing human population and increasing per capita use of water.

Water use in agriculture is of two kinds: irrigation of crops and watering of livestock. Many methods of crop irrigation are wasteful of water in that much of it is lost into the air by evaporation before it is taken up by crops. Livestock use

1 km$^3$ is the volume of a cube with 1 km sides. It is equivalent to 1 trillion litres or 10$^{12}$ litres.

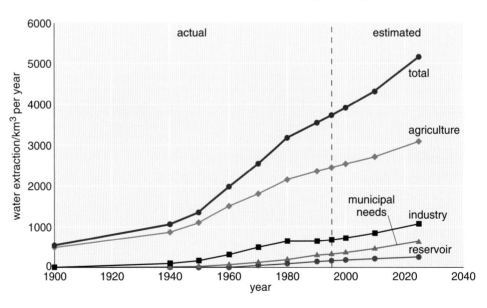

**Figure 3.5** Graph showing the amount of water extracted globally from natural reserves (rivers, lakes and groundwater) and used for four use categories. Water extraction is measured in cubic kilometres (km$^3$) per year. Data from 1900 to 1995 are actual figures; from 1995 to 2025 they are estimated. (Source: Houghton, 2004, Figure 7.6, p. 155)

**Table 3.2** Volume of water required to produce 1 kilogram (kg) of specific food products. (Source: data derived from UNESCO, 2003, Figure 1, p. 17)

| Product | Water required/litres |
|---|---|
| fresh meat – beef | 15 000 |
| fresh meat – lamb | 10 000 |
| poultry meat | 6000 |
| palm oil | 2000 |
| cereals | 1500 |
| citrus fruit | 1000 |
| pulses, roots and tubers | 1000 |

even more water. Table 3.2 compares the amounts of water required to produce various major food products. Notice how 'expensive' it is to produce beef and lamb in terms of water requirements.

The supply of clean water is affected by how people dispose of their waste water. People living in areas where there is no sanitation system for the disposal of waste water have little choice but to throw it away into a river or onto the ground. Each litre of water disposed of in this way pollutes an average of eight litres of freshwater, and the UN estimates that the global human population pollutes 12 000 km³ of water annually in this way. Unless there is major investment in sanitation systems, this figure will have increased to 18 000 km³ by 2050 (UNESCO, 2003).

### 3.3.1 The impact of climate change on global freshwater resources

The availability of freshwater will be significantly altered in a future world affected by climate change (Houghton, 2004). In some regions, water availability will decrease; in others it will increase. Precise predictions about the extent and exact location of such changes cannot be made, because they are based on climate models, the accuracy of which is uncertain. However, there is wide agreement that probable changes will include:

- More rain in northern high latitudes in winter and in the monsoon regions of south east Asia in summer.
- Less rain in southern Europe, Central America, southern Africa and Australia in summer.
- Greater water flows in rivers that are fed by glaciers.
- Overall, higher temperatures in all regions, which will lead to greater evaporation, so that, even in regions where rainfall does not decrease, water availability will be reduced.
- Rising sea levels, which will lead to flooding of low-lying coastal regions, including major flood plains and river deltas, many of which are currently densely populated; for example, the Bengal delta in Bangladesh contains 8.5 million people (Hecht, 2006) (see Figure 3.6).

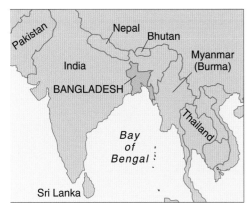

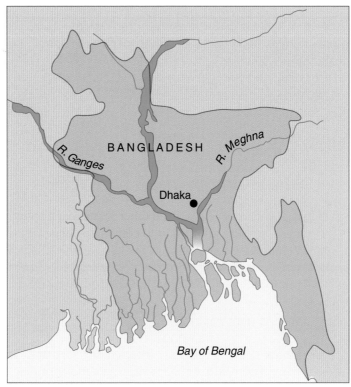

**Figure 3.6** Map of Bangladesh showing the extensive delta formed by the Rivers Ganges, Brahmaputra and Meghna.

The impact of Hurricane Katrina on the Mississippi delta in southern USA in 2005 revealed some of the adverse effects of human activities on river deltas. Control of water flow higher up-river reduces the amount of sediment reaching a delta, causing the land to subside. This is exacerbated by extraction of groundwater within the delta. Rising sea levels, resulting from climate change, may then threaten to inundate the lowered delta, especially during very severe weather (Hecht, 2006). In the Mississippi delta, the situation was exacerbated by inadequate maintenance of flood barriers.

As a result of the changes listed above, some regions will experience a greater frequency of flooding, while others will experience more frequent and more severe droughts. These changes will affect human health directly, as well as indirectly by disrupting agriculture and the supply of food.

The impending water crisis is bringing about a major change in the way that the water extraction industry approaches its task (Gleick, 2003). In the past, the emphasis was on finding more effective ways of extracting water from natural resources; now the emphasis is on finding more efficient ways to use it. For example, in California, considerable reductions in water use have been achieved. More efficient ways of irrigating farmland have been developed that decrease the amount of water lost by evaporation to the air. Domestic use of water has been reduced by the introduction of new designs of toilets, showers, washing machines and dishwashers. For example, domestic consumption of water to dispose of sewage in the USA has been reduced by 75% over 20 years by changes in toilet design. Similar reductions in domestic water use have been achieved in Australia, Japan and Europe (Gleick, 2003).

## 3.4 Water-borne infectious diseases

Water provides an environment for a huge variety of microbes, a small minority of which can cause disease in humans. Pathogenic microbes (Box 2.1) include viruses, bacteria, protoctists (proh-tok-tists) and larger creatures such as flukes and tapeworms. **Water-borne infectious diseases** are those in which the pathogen causing the disease lives part of its life cycle in water. Water-*associated* infectious diseases are those, like malaria, in which the animal that transmits the pathogen between people (mosquitoes) lives part of its life in water. To eliminate water-borne infectious diseases in a human population, two things have to be achieved. The first is a reliable supply of water that is not contaminated by pathogens. The second is an effective sanitation system that removes and disposes of human, animal and other waste that may be contaminated by pathogens, without allowing it to come into contact with the water supply. In developed countries, such as the UK and the USA, clean water and effective sanitation are available to virtually everyone. Nonetheless, occasionally one or other of these systems break down, even in the most technologically advanced countries, as will be described in Section 3.4.3. Such events are a salutary reminder that water is a very effective medium for spreading pathogens quickly and widely; a breakdown in either water or sanitation systems can lead to a very large number of people being infected in a very short time.

Protoctists are single-celled organisms which, until recently, biologists called protozoans

### 3.4.1 Diarrhoeal diseases

Freshwater habitats are home to two general types of human pathogen. First, there are those that are free-living in water, of which the bacterium that causes cholera is an example. Second, there are pathogens that live part of their lives in another freshwater animal, called a secondary host; *Schistosoma* (shist-oh-soh-ma), a microscopic fluke that lives in water snails, causes one such disease. The most common water-borne diseases are those that cause diarrhoea.

**Diarrhoeal diseases** are caused by a wide variety of pathogens, including viruses, bacteria and protoctists. Cholera is a diarrhoeal disease, caused by the bacterium *Vibrio cholerae*, and is discussed in detail in Section 3.4.2. Such pathogens infect the gut and irritate the cells lining its surface. The cells respond by secreting large amounts of water, and dissolved salts, into the gut which, in turn, responds by contracting to expel the watery, infected waste. If infection persists and causes prolonged and severe diarrhoea, water and body salts are lost in such large quantities that the chemistry of the whole body is disrupted.

The conventions for naming organisms in biology were given in Box 1.3.

◆ What other health-damaging effect do you think diarrhoea will have?

◆ Diarrhoeal infections also prevent the gut from breaking down and absorbing nutrients, causing malnutrition and increased susceptibility to other infections.

Even mild diarrhoeal infections are harmful to children if they persist, because they create a 'vicious cycle' of water loss and malnutrition that stunts their growth and development. You will recall that being underweight, as the result of malnutrition, is the leading global risk factor for poor health, as measured in DALYs (look back at Table 2.4). Until the 1950s, nutritional disorders and infectious diseases were generally regarded as quite distinct medical problems. Since then, however, the strong interaction between diarrhoeal diseases and nutrition has become much more widely recognised. In particular, much research has gone into explaining how malnutrition affects the immune system and lowers the body's ability to resist infection (Scrimshaw, 2003). **Immunodeficiency** is a condition in which the immune system fails to respond normally to an infection; it can be caused by a genetic defect and by HIV/AIDS, as well as by malnutrition. (The term is often confused with immunosuppression, which refers to the deliberate suppression of the immune system by means of drugs to prevent the rejection of transplanted organs.)

The treatment of diarrhoeal diseases is relatively simple, cheap and effective and consists of oral rehydration therapy (ORT). This involves drinking a solution that replenishes lost water and salts, and provides glucose for energy until the infection subsides (Figure 3.7). Despite the fact that ORT is simple and cheap, diarrhoeal diseases are a major cause of mortality, especially among children, in large parts of the world (Table 3.3). They are also a major cause of morbidity; many children under five years of age in developing regions of the world, experience several episodes of diarrhoea each year (Kosek et al., 2003).

As Table 3.3 shows, the impact of diarrhoeal diseases on child health is a huge problem in developing countries; even in Eastern Europe a total of 35 000 young children die from diarrhoeal diseases every year, representing 13% of all child deaths. By contrast, the extreme rarity of such deaths in wealthy developed nations reflects the disparity in the extent to which children have access to a reliable supply of clean water and a good sanitation system.

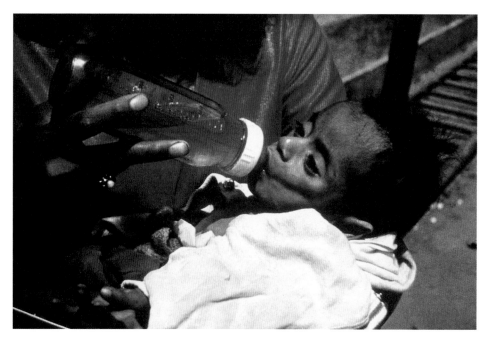

**Figure 3.7**   A baby suffering severe dehydration as a result of a diarrhoeal disease is given oral rehydration solution. (Photo: courtesy of Teaching Aids at Low Cost (TALC), PO Box 49, St Albans, UK. Details of TALC materials sent on request.)

**Table 3.3** Annual number of deaths among children under 5 years old due to diarrhoeal diseases in different world regions (as defined by the WHO) in the period 2000 to 2003, and the proportion of all deaths (the proportional mortality) among children under 5 due to this cause. (Source: data derived from WHO, 2005a, Statistical Annex, Table 3)

| Region | Africa | South East Asia | Western Pacific, excluding Australia, New Zealand, Japan | The Americas, excluding USA and Canada | Eastern Europe | USA, Canada, Western Europe, Israel, Australia, New Zealand, Japan | World |
|---|---|---|---|---|---|---|---|
| Number of deaths | 701 000 | 552 000 | 178 000 | 51 000 | 35 000 | 0 | 1 762 000 |
| Proportion of all deaths in this age group | 16% | 18% | 18% | 13% | 13% | 0% | 17% |

Table 3.4 compares the provision of water and sanitation in the UK with that of a number of African countries.

◆ Refer back to Table 2.1. Has global mortality due to diarrhoeal diseases changed since 1990?

◆ Yes, it has. In 1990 diarrhoeal diseases were ranked fourth among causes of mortality, responsible for 2.95 million deaths. In 2002, global mortality had fallen to 1.80 million, and their ranking had fallen to seventh.

Looking specifically at children, the total number dying from diarrhoeal diseases worldwide, referred to as the global burden of diarrhoeal disease, has been

**Table 3.4** Proportion of the human population with access to clean water and sanitation in the UK and four African countries in 2002. (Source: data derived from WHO, 2006, Annex Table 7)

| Country | Improved water source* | | Improved sanitation* | |
|---|---|---|---|---|
| | Urban | Rural | Urban | Rural |
| UK | 100% | 100% | 100% | 100% |
| South Africa | 98% | 73% | 86% | 44% |
| Ghana | 93% | 68% | 74% | 46% |
| Togo | 80% | 36% | 71% | 15% |
| Rwanda | 92% | 69% | 56% | 38% |

*The definitions of 'improved water source' and 'improved sanitation' used by the WHO are complex and relate to the type of technology used. Improved water sources involve technologies that provide clean, safe drinking water. Improved sanitation involves technologies that reduce direct human contact with excreta.

steadily declining, as water supplies and sanitation are slowly improved in developing countries (Figure 3.8). There has not, however, been a corresponding decline in morbidity; children who suffer from diarrhoea still average 3.2 episodes per year (Kosek et al., 2003). This suggests that there is an 'all-or none' effect, whereby fully improved water supplies and sanitation eliminate diarrhoeal diseases completely, but anything less than this exposes children to as much illness as no improvement at all. ORT reduces mortality by treating the *symptoms* of diarrhoea, but it does not prevent children from catching the disease.

WHO and UN data show a very strong association across different countries between the provision of clean water and effective sanitation, and death rates due to diarrhoeal diseases among young children; the poorer the provision, the higher the death rate.

### 3.4.2 Cholera

Whenever there is an environmental catastrophe, such as an earthquake or a major flood, there is usually the expectation that it will be followed by an epidemic of cholera. This indicates, first, that the pathogen that causes cholera, *Vibrio cholerae*, is widely present in the environment and, second, that epidemics are caused by damage to water and sanitation systems. On a global scale, the incidence of cholera has varied considerably during human history (look back at Figure 1.22). At present, humans are experiencing what is called the seventh pandemic, which began in 1961.

*Vibrio cholerae* is a bacterium with a wiggly tail, called a flagellum, that enables it to swim through water (Figure 3.9). It causes cholera only in humans, who become infected via drinking water and food, especially seafood. Cholera is an acute intestinal infection with a short incubation period, of between one and five days. The **incubation period** of a disease is the time between a pathogen entering its host and the host beginning to show disease symptoms. *Vibrio cholerae* attaches to the wall of the gut and produces a **toxin** that causes the cells in the gut wall to produces a copious, painless, watery diarrhoea that can quickly lead to severe dehydration and death if treatment is not promptly given. (A toxin is a poisonous substance produced by a living organism, usually injurious to potential prey, predators or competitors. Toxins are produced, not only by bacteria, but also by plants and animals.) Vomiting also occurs in most patients. However, most individuals infected with *V. cholerae* do not become ill, even though the bacterium is present in their faeces for 7–14 days.

◆ What are the implications of this for the spread of the disease?

◆ In the absence of proper sanitation, people infected with *V. cholerae* but not suffering from cholera symptoms, can none the less transmit *V. cholerae* to uninfected people, thus causing it to spread rapidly through a population.

When illness does occur, more than 90% of episodes are of mild or moderate severity and are difficult to distinguish clinically from other types of acute diarrhoea. Less than 10% of ill persons develop cholera with signs of moderate or severe dehydration. In those who do develop cholera, death occurs in 5 to 50%, depending on the effectiveness of the treatment that they receive.

If you are studying this book as part of an Open University course, go to Activity C3 in the *Companion* now.

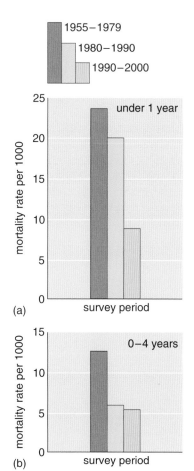

**Figure 3.8** Bar charts showing the results from two reviews of trends in child mortality due to diarrhoeal diseases in developing countries between 1955 and 2000. (Source: Kosek et al., 2003, p. 201)

The fact that relatively few of the people who become infected with *V. cholerae* develop full-blown cholera is related to the fact that cholera has a very high **infectious dose**. This is defined as the number of individual pathogens required to cause disease in an infected person. For cholera, the infectious dose is one hundred million bacteria. (For comparison, the infectious dose for malaria is just ten of the single-celled parasite that causes malaria.) In 'powers of ten' notation, one hundred million is written as $10^8$ (see Section 2.2.3 in the previous chapter).

There are many forms of *V. cholerae*, called strains, which show small genetic differences from one another, giving each strain slightly different properties. They are very abundant in both freshwater and seawater habitats, where they live attached to a variety of microscopic plants and animals (Gillespie and Bamford, 2000). Two strains, called O1 (also called El Tor) and O139, cause cholera in humans because they are able to make the powerful cholera toxin.

*Vibrio cholerae* thrives and reproduces in two quite distinct habitats: natural aquatic environments and human intestines (Cottingham et al., 2003). In essence, it is a common and harmless freshwater organism that sometimes infects people. This means that cholera presents a quite different challenge to health organisations, in comparison with diseases caused by pathogens that live only by infecting humans, such as measles or syphilis. There is much greater potential, at least in theory, to control and perhaps eliminate diseases such as measles altogether by such methods as vaccination and changing people's behaviour. It is much more difficult, if not impossible, to eliminate a pathogen that can live quite independently of humans, either in other animals, or, like cholera, in the natural environment. In nature, *V. cholerae* lives attached to other microscopic organisms; this opens a way to control cholera that has proved to be quite effective (see Section 3.4.4).

*Vibrio cholerae* is just as much at home in salt water as it is in freshwater and is becoming a major threat to people living and taking holidays in coastal communities. This is because rivers are becoming increasingly polluted, in particular with nitrates derived from fertilisers (see Section 3.6.2), and this pollution inevitably finds its way into the sea. There, it encourages the growth of huge blooms of algae, sometimes called 'red tides', which are being further encouraged by warmer seas, resulting from climate change. Algal blooms provide an ideal home for *V. cholerae*. The threat is particularly high in coastal communities where fish and other seafood represent a major component of the human diet (Epstein et al., 1993).

### 3.4.3 Cryptosporidiosis

Diarrhoeal diseases are not confined to the developing world. In the early spring of 1993, an outbreak of acute watery diarrhoea occurred in Milwaukee, USA, affecting 403 000 people, and killing 54 of them (MacKenzie et al., 1994; Furlow, 2005). The outbreak was due to a system failure at one of two water-treatment plants in the area, which enabled the single-celled (protoctist) parasite *Cryptosporidium* (Figure 3.10, overleaf) to pass through water filters and proliferate in the water supply. The disease caused by *Cryptosporidium* is called cryptosporidiosis (kript-oh-spor-id-ee-oh-sis).

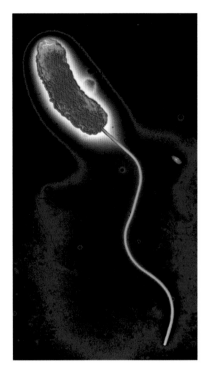

**Figure 3.9** A single *Vibrio cholerae* bacterium (often abbreviated to *V. cholerae*). The long tail, or flagellum, enables it to swim in water. Colours have been artificially added. Magnification · 10 000. (Photo: Eye of Science/Science Photo Library)

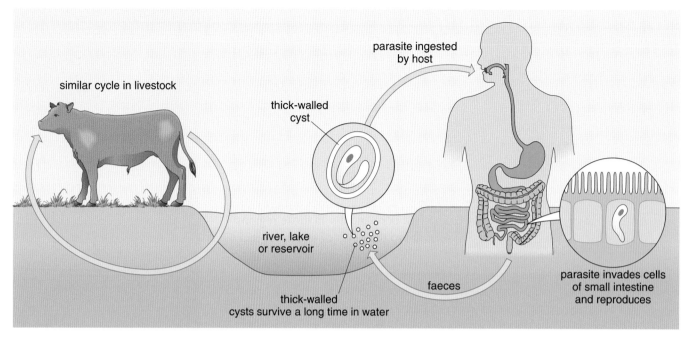

**Figure 3.10**    The life cycle of *Cryptosporidium*.

Outbreaks of cryptosporidiosis are quite common in developed countries such as the USA (Lee et al., 2002) and the UK, but are rarely such large-scale events as the 1993 outbreak in Milwaukee. A study of cryptosporidiosis outbreaks in England and Wales between 1989 and 1996 tested the hypothesis that outbreaks are associated with heavy rainfall, which can overload water-treatment plants (Lake et al., 2005). This association is rather weak, however, and it appears that the most common way by which *Cryptosporidium* gets into the water supply is from farm animals, pets and wildlife. *Cryptosporidium* has been found in untreated and treated drinking water supplies, swimming pools, rivers, streams and reservoirs in all parts of the world and is described as being ubiquitous (Meinhardt et al., 1996), meaning it is found everywhere.

Of the 54 people who died in the Milwaukee event, 46 had HIV/AIDS (Furlow, 2005). HIV attacks the immune system, reducing the capacity of the body to resist infection by pathogens.

◆  Can you recall what this phenomenon is called?

◆  Immunodeficiency (see Section 3.4.1).

The link between mortality due to cryptosporidiosis in Milwaukee and HIV/AIDS is a particular example of a more general problem that is particularly relevant in developing countries. Cryptosporidiosis, in common with other diarrhoeal diseases, is a disease that can cause morbidity in healthy people, but which can be fatal to people with a deficient immune system.

The link between malnutrition and immunodeficiency is very important in the context of this case study; it relates to the 'vicious cycle', mentioned in Section 3.4.1, involving malnutrition, diarrhoeal diseases and being underweight.

### 3.4.4 Preventing diarrhoeal diseases

Kibera is a huge shanty town in Nairobi, Kenya, which lacks an adequate water supply and sanitation (Figure 3.11). The health problems that affect people in Kibera occur in many parts of the developing world. An estimated 2.6 billion people globally have no access to even a simple pit latrine, and over one billion have no source of safe drinking water (Watkins, 2006). In such conditions, people are very vulnerable to infection by a range of water-borne infectious diseases, such as those discussed above.

It is possible to vaccinate people against cholera, but this protects them only for three to six months. Consequently, while vaccination is useful for protecting people who are visiting regions where cholera is prevalent, it does not provide a satisfactory means of control for people who live permanently in those regions. Certain features of *Cryptosporidium* are relevant to the kinds of strategies that *are* effective in controlling it. In contrast to *V. cholerae*, *Cryptosporidium* has a *low* infectious dose.

◈ Can you recall what this means?

◆ It means that infection with only a few organisms is enough to cause illness.

The infectious dose of *Cryptosporidium* is less than 10. The significance of this is that only water from which *all* pathogens have been removed is completely safe for human consumption. Removal of many kinds of pathogens from drinking water is achieved by the use of **disinfectant** chemicals in water treatment plants. (A disinfectant is a chemical that reduces microbial contamination of water, surfaces, etc.) However, at least one species of *Cryptosporidium*, called *C. parvum*, is naturally resistant to most chemical disinfectants (Gillespie and

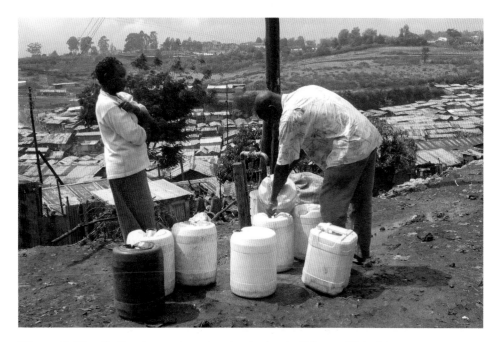

**Figure 3.11**   Collecting water at a stand-pipe in Kibera, Nairobi. (Photo: Jo Halliday).

Bamford, 2000). Ozone (a poisonous gas that occurs naturally high up in the atmosphere) is being increasingly used in sewage treatment plants to eliminate *Cryptosporidium*; this is not a perfect solution, as it can lead to high levels of bromate in drinking water. Bromate is a toxic substance that can cause cancer. (A well-known soft-drink company once had to withdraw its bottled water from the market in a country because of high bromate levels.)

A very simple and inexpensive method of combating cholera exploits the fact that, when living in water, *V. cholerae* lives attached to microscopic animals (zooplankton) and plants (phytoplankton). Though very small, these organisms are larger than *V. cholerae* and can be removed from water by fine-mesh filters, made of sari cloth or nylon (as you will see in DVD Activity 3.1). Use of such filters in 65 villages in rural Bangladesh between 1999 and 2002 led to a 48% reduction in the incidence of cholera (Colwell et al., 2003).

Filtering water in this way is called a **'point-of-use' strategy** for controlling disease. It depends on individual people treating water as they use it, rather than having purified water delivered to them from a remote water-treatment plant in pipes. Sachets of purification agents are increasingly being used as a point-of use strategy for making water safe to drink in regions of the world where water is not treated in large-scale plants before it is distributed (Lougheed, 2006) (Figure 3.12 and Activity 3.1).

### Water treatment: a difficult trade-off

The fact that people with deficient immune systems are more susceptible to water-borne pathogens such as *Cryptosporidium* takes us into a rather

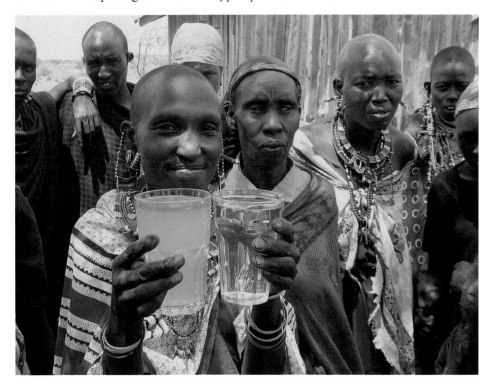

**Figure 3.12**  A Maasai woman in Kenya with glasses of water before and after simple purification treatment. (Photo: Greg Allgood/Procter and Gamble)

controversial area, which revolves around the question: is it sensible to seek to make drinking water *completely* free of pathogenic microbes? On the face of it, the answer would seem to be 'yes', but there are two reasons why it might not be desirable. First, complete elimination of microbes requires the use of very high levels of chemicals, some of which, like ozone, produce products that are themselves harmful to human health. Second, if people's immune systems are not occasionally exposed to a particular pathogen, they will not develop immunity to it. Thus, it is argued that it is no bad thing if drinking water contains pathogenic microbes at very low levels. Evidence in support of this comes from detailed studies following cryptosporidiosis outbreaks. People who live in areas where the water supply comes from surface sources, such as rivers and lakes, that are typically contaminated by *Cryptosporidium* from livestock, are less severely affected during cryptosporidiosis outbreaks than people whose water supply comes from deep, groundwater sources, which are not contaminated (Furlow, 2005).

## 3.5  Water chemistry and life

Water is by far the most abundant component of plants and animals: 60% of the human body is water. Life probably originated in water, many plants and animals live in it, and all the chemical reactions that take place in plant and animal bodies take place in water. The importance of water as a medium for life comes first from its abundance on Earth and second because it possesses five distinctive properties: its solvent properties; heat capacity; surface tension; freezing properties; and transparency. You will now examine each of these properties in turn.

### 3.5.1 The properties of water

On Earth, water is a liquid between 0 °C and 100 °C. If the Earth were as close to the Sun as Venus is, water would exist only as a gas; if the Earth were as far from the Sun as Mars is, water would be present only as ice. Water is a **chemical compound** made of **molecules** with the formula $H_2O$ (see Box 3.1). This tells you that each molecule is composed of two hydrogen **atoms** (H is the symbol used to denote the **element** hydrogen) and one oxygen atom (O is the symbol used to denote the element oxygen) (Figure 3.13). You will shortly learn more about atoms, molecules, elements and compounds and how they relate to the molecular structure of water in Activity 3.1 on the DVD associated with this book. The activity then goes on to deal with **ions** (eye-ons).

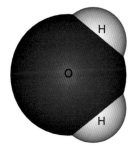

**Figure 3.13**  Model of a molecule of water consisting of one oxygen atom (O) joined to two hydrogen atoms (H). In molecular models such as these, it is the convention to use standard colours to symbolise atoms of different elements: hydrogen is white and oxygen is red, as here. Water molecules are extremely small (of the order $10^{10}$ m across), which is why models are used to visualise their behaviour.

---

**Box 3.1**  (Explanation) Definitions of some basic chemical terms

An **atom** is the smallest unit of an element that still has the properties of the element.

A **molecule** is two or more atoms held together by chemical bonds.

An **element** is a substance that cannot be broken down into a simpler substance; it is composed of just one type of atom.

An **ion** is an electrically charged atom or molecule.

A **chemical compound** is a substance made up of two or more elements; it may be composed of molecules or ions.

Water is a very good **solvent** in its liquid form, meaning that it is able to dissolve a wide range of substances. When you add salt to a pan of hot water, it quickly disappears; you have made a solution of salt in water. A liquid that dissolves another substance is called a solvent, and water is a solvent for many substances, including solids, such as salt, and gases, such as oxygen and carbon dioxide. As you will shortly learn in Activity 3.1 on the DVD associated with this book, its properties as a solvent stem from the fact that water is a **polar molecule**. The water molecule is said to be polar because it has negatively and positively charged regions, with the oxygen atom being slightly negatively charged and the hydrogen atoms slightly positively charged. You will see why this is important in Activity 3.1.

---

### Activity 3.1   Water, molecules and ions

Allow 1 hour for this activity

Now would be the ideal time to study the DVD activity entitled 'Water, molecules and ions' which you will find on the DVD associated with this book. The first part of the activity deals with the representation of molecules and what liquid water looks like at the molecular level, and in so doing covers some aspects of scale. The sequence begins by exploring in more detail the story of water contaminated with *Vibrio cholerae*. In order to understand how filtration works as a method of removing the bacteria it is necessary to examine the relative sizes of the mesh in sari cloth and the cholera bacteria. This provides practice in understanding relative scales and expressing very small distances in metres (the SI unit of length) and their subunits. Further magnification, this time using models, allows the nature of liquid water at the molecular level to be explored. After studying this part of the activity, you should have a better understanding of the relationship between the properties of liquid water on a macroscopic scale (water as you normally see it) and its molecular structure.

The DVD then goes on to examine the composition of an **ionic compound**, common salt (sodium chloride), and the process involved when ionic compounds dissolve in water. Finally it looks at other types of ion present in mineral water using molecular models. After playing this concluding part of the sequence, you should have a better understanding of the nature of some of the dissolved ions, both harmless and potentially harmful, commonly found in water.

If you are unable to play this sequence now, try to do so as soon as possible. You will find it harder to study the rest of this chapter until you have done so.

---

As Activity 3.1 demonstrated, it is its polar properties that make water such a good solvent. Take common salt as an example (Figure 3.14a). The chemical name for common salt is sodium chloride and its formula is NaCl (en-aye-see-ell). Here Na is the symbol for the element sodium (from the Latin name *natrium*) and Cl is the symbol for the element chlorine. Sodium chloride is not made up of molecules, like water is. Instead it is made up of ions, which are electrically charged, in this case sodium ions (denoted Na$^+$) and chloride ions (denoted Cl$^-$). (Note the slight change of name from chlorine (the element) to chloride (the ion), which is the convention used by scientists.) In a crystal of common salt

(Figure 3.14a), the sodium ions and chloride ions are in a regular arrangement (Figure 3.14b) held together by the attraction between the opposite charges.

When added to water, common salt quickly dissolves. This involves the attractive forces within the crystal being replaced by attractive forces between water molecules and the individual $Na^+$ and $Cl^-$ ions (Figure 3.15).

Many biologically important substances, such as amino acids (ah-meen-oh acids, the building blocks of which proteins are made) or sugars (for example glucose,

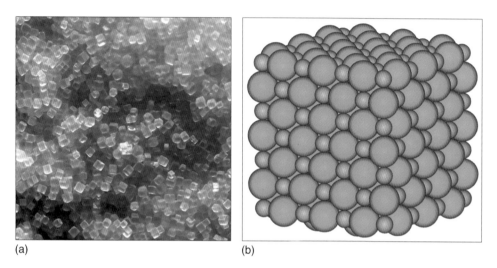

(a)　　　　　　　　　　　　　　　　(b)

**Figure 3.14** (a) Crystals of common salt, sodium chloride (magnified) (Photo: Diane Diederich/istockphoto). (b) Model of the arrangement of positively charged sodium ions (silver) and negatively charged chloride ions (green) in sodium chloride crystals.

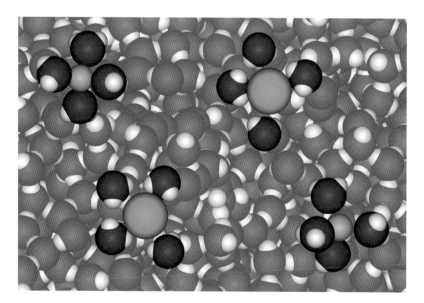

**Figure 3.15** Salt (sodium chloride) dissolved in water. The negatively charged oxygen atoms (red) are attracted to the positively charged sodium ions (silver) and the positively charged hydrogen atoms (white) are attracted to the negatively charged chloride ions (green). The background water molecules are shown paler for clarity.

fructose or sucrose found in foods), are made of molecules, not charged ions, but none the less they dissolve readily in water. That is because, like water, they are polar molecules with positively and negatively charged regions that are respectively attracted to the negatively and positively charged regions of water molecules.

Water has other important properties. It has a high **heat capacity**, meaning that it requires more energy to raise its temperature by 1 °C than it does to heat up, say, air or a rock by the same amount. This means that water maintains a more stable temperature than the air or rocks in the face of variations in the temperature of the environment. Most of the chemical reactions involved in life processes can only occur over a narrow range of temperatures, so it is important that the temperature of animals and plants does not vary too much.

Water also has a high *surface tension* that creates a distinct surface layer at the interface between water and air. This is a consequence of the network of **hydrogen bonds** between water molecules, which were described in Activity 3.1. The high surface tension enables animals such as pond skaters to scoot about on its surface, and (for complex reasons that we don't have space to explain) enables trees to be very tall.

Most liquids become more dense (i.e. they compress, become smaller) as they cool but water, most unusually, becomes more dense down to 4 °C, but then *expands* between 4 °C and 0 °C. As a result at 0 °C, ice is *less* dense than liquid water. It therefore forms on the surface of water, enabling plants and animals to survive cold weather beneath the ice. This is another consequence of the network of hydrogen bonds between water molecules.

Finally, the transparency of water means that sunlight can pass through it, enabling plants to grow in it, supporting complex communities of animals.

Of these properties of water, the most significant in the context of this chapter is that chemical compounds dissolve in it. Also important is the fact that, as water circulates around the global environment, it sometimes exists as a solid (ice), and sometimes as a gas (water vapour), as well as in its liquid form.

### 3.5.2 Pure water or clean water?

No natural water found on Earth is pure; rainwater is very nearly pure, but contains dissolved gases such as oxygen and carbon dioxide from the atmosphere. Water does not need to be pure to be acceptable for human consumption; indeed, the fashion for 'natural' spring water is evidence for the value people place on certain dissolved minerals. The label on a bottle of mineral water lists all the dissolved substances, such as calcium, many of them very good for you, which it contains. Accordingly, to distinguish water that is safe to drink from that which is not, rather than describing it inaccurately as 'pure', the term 'clean' is used.

Absolutely pure water would not support life and it is the many and varied substances that become dissolved in water that make it a medium in which microbes can live and reproduce. Most microbes present no threat to the health of humans and other organisms, but are engaged in thoroughly useful activities, such as breaking down potentially toxic waste and converting poisonous substances into safe ones. Only a tiny minority of microbes are harmful to the health of other organisms such as those you have already read about in Section 3.4.

Water purity is a relative concept and no system for providing water to human populations aims to deliver absolutely pure water. Rather, national or international authorities try to supply clean water by establishing standards for water quality that specify the maximum amounts of microbes and of various harmful chemicals that are considered acceptable in the water supplied for human consumption.

## 3.6    Chemical pollution of water

Toxic substances are a feature of the natural world; many plants contain chemical compounds that make them anything from mildly distasteful to lethally poisonous to animals that might eat them. Some animals are equipped to deal with dangerous plants in their environment and possess detoxification mechanisms that break down harmful compounds. Humans, for example, rely on their liver to neutralise the harmful effects of alcohol. During human cultural evolution, cooking techniques have developed that destroy toxic chemicals in plants. Examples include nerve poisons in the lentils from which dahl is made in India, and cyanide in cassava, a staple crop in Africa and South America. There are limits, however, to what the liver and cooking can achieve and the environment contains a huge array of chemical compounds, some of them of human manufacture, that are harmful to human health and survival. The latter are said to be **xenobiotic** (zen-oh-bye-ot-ik). Literally meaning 'alien to nature', in the context of this book this word refers to chemicals 'of human origin'.

The harmful effects of alcohol are discussed in another book in this series (Smart, 2007)

Water is said to be polluted, or contaminated, whenever any harmful or undesirable change in its physical, chemical or biological quality results from the release into it of synthetic or naturally occurring chemicals, radioactivity or **organic** matter. (Organic means arising from the bodies of plants, animals or other organisms.) Pollution often refers to the results of human activity but there are significant natural causes of contamination, such as volcanic eruptions, which release a variety of chemicals, and tsunamis, which mix salty seawater with freshwater. Much of the groundwater obtained from boreholes in parts of Bangladesh and West Bengal is contaminated with naturally-occurring arsenic, released from rocks deep underground.

Contamination can occur at many points in the global water cycle depicted in Figure 3.3. Most familiarly, pollutants can be released into rivers or into the sea, but they can also be released into groundwater by pollution of the soil. Some pollutants enter the water cycle from the atmosphere; for example, acid rain is caused by the mixing of water vapour with gaseous pollutants such as sulfur dioxide, released by burning fossil fuels, and a variety of nitrogen compounds, from agricultural fertilisers (see Section 3.6.3).

Sulfur dioxide has the chemical formula $SO_2$ (one atom of sulfur, two atoms of oxygen); some texts still use the older spelling 'sulphur'.

Pollution may be acute or chronic. *Acute pollution* events refer to the sudden release of large quantities of a contaminant, usually leading to very obvious harmful effects. An example is provided by the accidental release of a large quantity of aluminium sulfate, a substance used in water treatment, into the water supply of Camelford, in Cornwall in July 1988, leading to severe loss of mental

Acute and chronic diseases and health conditions were defined in Section 1.6.1.

function in a large number of people (Altmann et al., 1999). *Chronic pollution* refers to the slow and persistent contamination of water through the sustained release of a pollutant and is, in many ways, a more serious concern, for three reasons. Chronic pollution may go undetected for a long time; it is generally more difficult to rectify than an acute pollution event; chronic pollution is also serious because, unlike most acute pollution events, it is often not confined, as the Camelford tragedy was, to a small area.

One of the most toxic of xenobiotic pollutants, dioxin, formed by the burning of plastics and certain fertilisers, has become ubiquitous (found everywhere) and can be detected in virtually every person that has been tested for it throughout the world (Sargent, 2005).

As a result of the risks arising from pollution, the water supply in high-income countries is carefully monitored to ensure that levels of contaminants do not exceed specified concentrations that are considered to be safe. The determination of safe levels is quite a complex process that involves the science of **toxicology** (the study of toxins and their effects on living organisms). This involves exposing animals to a toxic compound, to determine its lethal dose. Among the animals used for toxicological testing of water-borne chemicals are tadpoles of the African clawed frog (*Xenopus laevis*) (Figure 3.16). *Xenopus* is widely used for this purpose as it breeds readily in captivity and produces huge numbers of tadpoles. Recall that frogs and amphibians are regarded as particularly sensitive indicators of environmental damage (Box 1.1).

There is growing recognition that determining the lethal dose of a compound in *Xenopus* tadpoles in a laboratory is not very helpful in trying to determine if that compound poses a threat to human health.

◆ Why do you suppose this is?

◆ For a start, there is the question of whether *Xenopus* is more or less sensitive to the compound than humans. Furthermore, the lethal dose approach is a measurement only of mortality, and provides no information about morbidity.

Another approach to the study of pollution is the science of **ecotoxicology**, which is the study of the fate of contaminants in the natural environment and of their effects on plants, animals and **ecosystems**. (Ecosystems are recognisable assemblages of plants and animals, such as woodland, grassland, rivers, etc., in which a distinct set of plants and animals live together and interact with one another.) This asks, not how much of a compound does it take to kill a tadpole, but what is the effect on a tadpole of the compound at the kind of concentration that occurs in the wild?

Much environmental damage has been done in Scandinavia by acid rain caused by industrial pollution from the industrial north of Britain, swept across the North Sea by the prevailing wind. For example, populations of frogs and newts have declined widely and disappeared altogether in some localities. If frog tadpoles are reared in water that is acidified to the same level as Scandinavian pond water, they do not die. Rather, they become lethargic and feed less than tadpoles in non-acidified water (Griffiths et al., 1994). They do not grow as fast as healthy tadpoles; they later become under-sized frogs and they do not survive to breed.

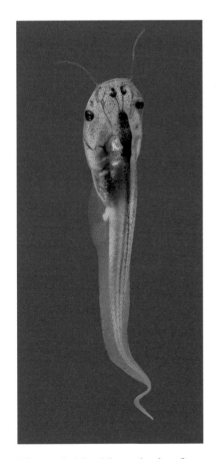

**Figure 3.16**  The tadpole of *Xenopus laevis*. (Photo: Ronn Altig)

The result is the same as if tadpoles dropped dead when exposed to acid water; the frog population declines. By focusing on often very subtle, non-lethal effects of pollutants, ecotoxicologists provide a more complete and precise assessment of how pollutants affect wildlife than can be derived by determining their lethal dose. If it seems odd to you that scientists study the possible human health effects of xenobiotic chemicals by looking at their effects on tadpoles, bear in mind that it would be impossible, for ethical reasons, to test the effects of such chemicals on humans directly.

*Bioaccumulation*

When chemical contaminants enter the body of a person, they circulate around the body in the blood. Different contaminants have different chemical properties and specific contaminants tend to accumulate in specific parts of the body, called target tissues, or in substances produced in the body such as breast milk (Table 3.5).

**Table 3.5** Some common pollutants and their target tissues. (Source: data derived from Connell et al., 1999, Table 4.1, p. 55)

| Pollutant | Target tissues or substances |
| --- | --- |
| lead | bone, teeth, nervous tissue |
| mercury | nervous tissue, particularly the brain |
| organochlorine pesticides, polychlorinated biphenyls (PCBs) | fatty tissue, breast milk |
| asbestos | lungs |

The affinity of specific pollutants for specific target tissues is related to a very important aspect of ecotoxicology, called **bioaccumulation**. This refers to the fact that, having been released into the environment, a pollutant is not randomly or evenly dispersed, but becomes concentrated into particular components of ecosystems. For example, DDT is accumulated in the fat reserves of birds, where it can reach quite high levels. (DDT, dichloro-diphenyl-trichloroethane, was the first widely used synthetic pesticide and has been used to kill agricultural and domestic insect pests since 1939; see Section 3.6.1.) This has two important effects. In the affected bird, it means that, if it uses its fat reserves to provide energy for some specific activity, such as reproduction or migration, a large dose of DDT is released into its blood over a short time. Every time a predator eats such a bird, it too receives a large dose which, in turn, is stored in its fat. The consequence of bioaccumulation is that contaminants that may be quite safe to wildlife, or humans, when encountered at the kind of concentrations at which they are released into water, can become concentrated at particular points in the food-chain, at levels that are not safe (Figure 3.17, overleaf).

## 3.6.1  DDT: a classic case in ecotoxicology

DDT is very effective in controlling pests, being very toxic to insects, and cheap to produce. Its effectiveness is enhanced because it is very persistent,

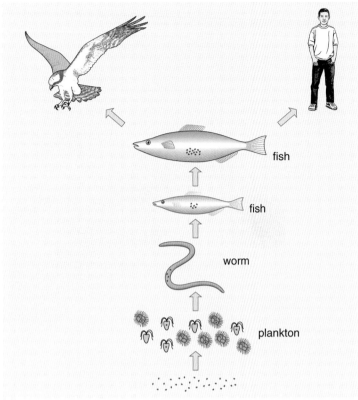

| location | DDT concentration/ppm | |
|---|---|---|
| | decimal | powers of ten |
| humans | 6.0 | |
| fish (freshwater) | 2.0 | |
| fish (marine) | 0.5 | $5 \times 10^{-1}$ |
| aquatic invertebrates (freshwater and marine) | 0.1 | $10^{-1}$ |
| freshwater | 0.00001 | $10^{-5}$ |
| seawater | 0.000001 | $10^{-6}$ |

(b)

(a)

**Figure 3.17** (a) Diagram showing bioaccumulation of a chemical contaminant in an aquatic food-chain. (b) Concentrations of DDT (in ppm, parts per million) in different parts of the environment. (Source: data derived from Freedman, 1989)

remaining active in the environment for a long time. This increases its value as an insecticide to farmers, because one application lasts a long time, but is also a major reason why it poses a threat to wildlife and to human health. Although the agricultural use of DDT was banned in most developed countries 30 years ago, it can still be detected in samples taken from the soil, from water and from the bodies of animals; it is also detectable in people.

Concern about the widespread effects of DDT led to it being banned in most developed countries in the 1960s and 1970s, but it is still used extensively in many developing countries, not least because it is very effective at controlling disease-carrying insects. DDT is credited with having eliminated malaria from Europe and the USA. The WHO has recently agreed that the human health benefits of using DDT in malaria areas outweigh the environmental risks, and it is a front-line weapon against the mosquitoes that carry malaria. Efforts are being made, however, to reduce the quantities used; for example, DDT-impregnated bed nets are increasingly been used instead of spraying (Figure 3.18).

The harmful effects of DDT on wildlife were first detected in 1947, when dramatic declines in a number of birds of prey, particularly the peregrine falcon, were noted in Britain. Similar declines were detected in the USA, especially among birds such as ospreys that eat fish. By the early 1960s the link between such declines and DDT had been worked out.

◆ Why are birds like ospreys and peregrine falcons at particular risk?

◆ Peregrines and ospreys prey on mammals and fish and so occupy a position at the top of food-chains, in which DDT-affected insects occupy a low level so that, through bioaccumulation, they build up DDT in high concentrations in their body fat.

The most severely poisoned birds died; those that did not die produced eggs with shells so thin that they collapsed under the weight of the parents in the nest. The use of the breeding birds' fat reserves during egg production released large amounts of DDT, affecting the deposition of calcium in egg shells. This is an example of a phenomenon called endocrine disruption (see Section 3.6.4).

DDT has been suggested as a causal factor for a number of human health problems. Detailed studies have ruled out a suggested link between DDT and breast cancer, but it is still strongly suspected to be linked to pancreatic cancer, neuropsychological dysfunction and some reproductive problems (Beard, 2006).

DDT is only one of a vast array of pesticides that is now in use. In 1995, 2.6 million metric tons of active pesticide ingredients, worth $38 billion, were used around the world (WRI, 1999). 85% of this was used in agriculture, much of which produces crops in developing countries, such as cotton, bananas, coffee, vegetables and flowers, that are exported to developed countries. In 2000, an estimated 3.75 million metric tons were manufactured worldwide; on current trends, global pesticide production is predicted to reach 6.55 million metric tons in 2025 and 10.1 million in 2050 (Tilman et al., 2001).

## 3.6.2 Mercury

Mercury is a naturally occurring metal which, in its pure form, is not particularly toxic. Under normal conditions of temperature and pressure, it is a silvery-white liquid which readily transforms into a vapour. When vaporised, it enters the atmosphere, remains there for a long time, and is circulated globally (WHO 2005b). Through chemical reaction and precipitation it enters freshwater lakes and rivers, where it accumulates in the sediments at the bottom. Here it is transformed by bacteria into a variety of mercury compounds, particularly methyl mercury (chemical formula: $CH_3Hg^+$) which is highly toxic. From freshwater sediments methyl mercury is taken up by small organisms and enters aquatic food chains, accumulating in the fat of animals and, by bioaccumulation, reaching high levels in animals towards the top of the food-chain, such as larger fish and fish-eating birds (Zahir et al., 2005).

The realisation that mercury compounds pose a serious threat to human health began with an unfolding tragedy in Minamata Bay, Japan, beginning in the mid-1950s (Connell et al., 1999). As is often the case, the first evidence that something was amiss came from observations of animals. Birds flew erratically and sometimes fell into the sea; children were able to catch usually evasive octopuses with their bare hands; cats had convulsions and died. It was not until the 1960s that many local people became overtly ill. They had convulsions, began to stagger about and salivated excessively; deaths began to occur,

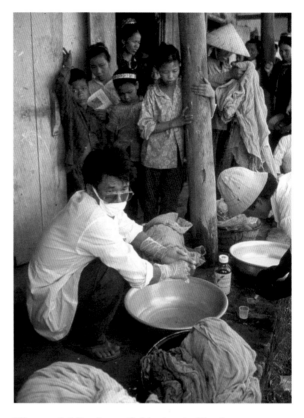

**Figure 3.18** Insecticide-treated bed nets have to be re-treated regularly. Communal 'dipping' sessions, here in Viet Nam, encourage community participation and have reduced the incidence of malaria by up to 50% in some areas. (Photo: WHO/TDR/Martel)

The chemical symbol for the element mercury is Hg, which derives from its ancient name *hydrargyrum*, meaning 'liquid silver'.

including newly-born children. The source of the problem was a chemical factory that was discharging its waste into Minamata Bay. This waste included large amounts of methyl mercury, estimated at 600 tons between 1932 and 1970. The animals and the people were suffering from mercury poisoning, now sometimes called 'Minamata disease'.

The principal sources of atmospheric mercury are the burning of fossil fuels in power stations and of domestic and industrial wastes in incinerators. Mercury compounds are also released directly to the land in many fungicides (chemicals used to protect crops from fungal diseases) (Clean Air Network, 1999). Mercury compounds have been used as an ingredient of some cosmetics, and even some vaccines. A compound of mercury called thiomersal in the UK (or thimerosal in the USA) has been used as a preservative in vaccines since 1931. In the late 1990s, some safety concerns about thiomersal led to its gradual withdrawal from some of the vaccines in which it had been an ingredient (note: it was never used in the measles, mumps and rubella MMR vaccine in the UK), but a WHO expert committee concluded that there is no evidence of any toxicity and it remains in use (GACVS, 2006).

### The effects of mercury compounds on wildlife and on people

Mercury compounds have no effect on plants, but adverse effects have been demonstrated in a wide range of animals, including fish and amphibians (Boening, 2000). Very high levels of mercury have been found in the livers of American alligators in the severely polluted Everglades of Florida; these can be as much as 400 times greater than levels in alligators born and reared in alligator farms (Linder and Grillitsch, 2000).

◆ By what process would such high levels of mercury arise in alligators?

◆ Bioaccumulation. Alligators are large, predatory animals that feed on fish.

Methyl mercury pollution is implicated in the near extinction of populations of stream-living salamanders in Acadia National Park, Maine (Bank et al., 2006).

The most important effect that mercury compounds have on people is on children born to women exposed to high levels during pregnancy (WHO, 2004). In extreme cases they have seizures and cerebral palsy; they may also be born blind or deaf. In less extreme cases, they have reduced intelligence, poor memory, and attention deficit disorder. Mercury compounds have no detectable effect on the mother, but can be detected in her hair, and mercury levels in maternal hair are strongly related to the severity of post-birth effects in children (Cohen et al., 2005).

Infants can also be exposed to mercury compounds via breast-milk. In some fishing communities the concentration of mercury in children's hair is correlated with the duration of breast-feeding. Reports of high mercury levels in mothers and children mostly come from regions where people eat a lot of fish; for example, high levels of blood mercury have been detected in people in the USA who identify themselves as Asians, Pacific Islanders, or Native Americans (Hightower et al., 2006). The unsaturated fats that occur in fish have beneficial consequences for human health and people are encouraged to eat fish in many countries. Currently, the US government encourages the eating of fish in the general population, but discourages it in women of childbearing age because of the risk posed to unborn children by mercury compounds (Cohen et al., 2005). Around the Faeroe Islands especially high levels of mercury have been found in pilot whales and, as a consequence, pregnant women are encouraged to avoid eating whale meat (Booth and Zeller, 2005).

Mercury compounds represent a major threat to human health in the future. Mercury emissions from power stations and other sources are not controlled in most countries. For example, at the time of writing in 2006 they were not covered by US Clean Air legislation (Clean Air Network, 1999). The rate of emissions has been increasing; there was a 10% increase in the USA from 2001 to 2002, and, in countries such as China and India, whose rapidly expanding economies are heavily dependent on fossil fuels, emissions are predicted to increase even faster (Booth and Zeller, 2005). The effects of mercury pollution will be global; because mercury can be dispersed as a vapour it can be deposited anywhere in the world.

Current inaction over mercury contrasts strongly with what has happened in relation to another toxic metal, lead. Lead is recognised as a very important toxin for children (WHO, 2004). Like mercury, it has serious effects on the developing nervous system, causing impaired brain function, leading, for example, to attention deficit disorder. In many high-income countries, the most obvious sources of lead have been eliminated; lead is no longer used for water pipes, and has been removed from petrol and paint. Lead has long been subject to a surveillance programme in the USA, but no such programme yet exists for mercury (Schweiger, 2005).

### 3.6.3 Nitrogen: a developing threat to health

A great deal of attention, by governments and the media, is focused on the environmental threat posed by carbon dioxide ($CO_2$) emissions, and on the urgent need to reduce them. Mainly due to the burning of fossil fuels, the level of $CO_2$ in the atmosphere has increased by some 36% since pre-industrial times. According to recent estimates (IPCC, 2007), this increase has contributed more than 50% of the global warming attributed to human activities. The rest is due to enhanced atmospheric concentrations of a number of other 'greenhouse' gases, including nitrous oxide ($N_2O$). Molecule for molecule, $N_2O$ is nearly 300 times more powerful as a greenhouse gas than $CO_2$ and levels of the gas are rising rapidly, largely due to the widespread use of nitrogen fertilisers in agriculture; some of the nitrogen ends up in the air as $N_2O$. However, the amount of $N_2O$ in the atmosphere is still very low, and the observed increase (up 18% above pre-industrial level) has contributed just 5% to global warming *so far*.

Nitrogen exists in the environment in huge quantities; as nitrogen gas ($N_2$) it makes up 78% by volume of the Earth's atmosphere. As an element, nitrogen is an inert gas; that is, it is unreactive, is of little use to animals or plants and does no harm to them. It is when nitrogen becomes incorporated into compounds with other elements (notably oxygen or hydrogen) that it becomes reactive and can be harmful. In a natural environment, like that which existed before the industrial revolution, reactive compounds of nitrogen are produced naturally, in relatively small quantities. For example, lightning converts nitrogen in the atmosphere into compounds called *nitrates* that enter the soil in rain. Bacteria that occur in nodules on the roots of certain plants, known as nitrogen-fixing bacteria, also convert nitrogen gas into nitrogen compounds which enter the soil, providing a natural fertiliser.

The situation changed during the industrial revolution, with the burning of fossil fuels on a large scale, releasing various nitrogen compounds into the atmosphere in large quantities. More recently, the industrial production of nitrogen fertilisers has released into the environment a number of other, reactive nitrogen compounds. These are listed, with their effects, in Table 3.6 in Box 3.2.

The major source of nitrogen compounds in the environment is now the increasing use of fertilisers to enhance crop yields, driven largely by the need to feed the large proportion of the world's human population that is undernourished. This is a trend that is expected to continue (Figure 3.19).

Other sources of nitrogen being added to the environment are urine and manure from livestock, industrial emissions and human waste. As a result of all this release of nitrogen compounds, the natural cycle of nitrogen in the environment has become swamped by what is called the 'nitrogen cascade'

---

**Box 3.2** (Enrichment) Reactive compounds of nitrogen and their environmental effects

There are many compounds of nitrogen and they have a variety of effects on the environment. Table 3.6 lists a selection. The chemical formulae are included for completeness.

**Table 3.6**  Some compounds of nitrogen and their environmental effects. (Source: Hooper, 2006, p. 42)

| Compound | Chemical formulae | Environmental effects |
|---|---|---|
| nitrate ion[*] | $NO_3^-$ | acid rain, eutrophication of water[‡] |
| nitric acid | $HNO_3$ | acid rain, eutrophication of water |
| nitrogen dioxide | $NO_2$ | smog, acid rain, eutrophication of water |
| nitrous acid | $HNO_2$ | smog, acid rain |
| nitric oxide | $NO$ | smog, acid rain |
| nitrous oxide | $N_2O$ | greenhouse gas, destruction of ozone in the stratosphere |
| ammonia/ ammonium ion[*] | $NH_3/NH_4^+$ | smog, eutrophication of water, aerosols[§] |

[*]Recall from Activity 3.1 that these are polyatomic ions, since they contain several atoms joined together and they carry a positive or negative charge.

[‡]The term 'eutrophication of water' refers to the effect of high levels of nitrogen compounds in water; these include a reduction in biodiversity as the water becomes choked with algae.

[§]'Aerosols' refer to the formation of tiny particles, suspended in the atmosphere.

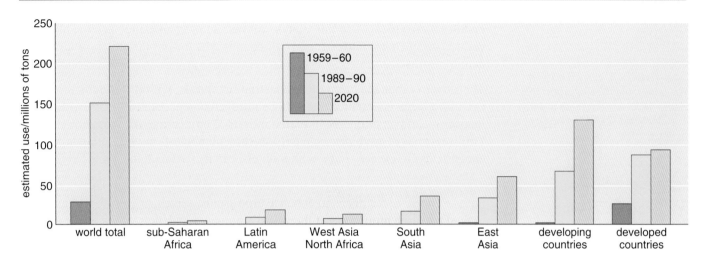

**Figure 3.19** Estimated growth in fertiliser use, 1959–2020. (Source: Bumb and Baanante, 1996, Table 1)

(Galloway et al., 2003). In the natural nitrogen cycle (Figure 3.20), *de-nitrifying* bacteria convert nitrogen compounds back into atmospheric nitrogen, but these are now unable to cope with the massive quantities currently being released into the environment. As a result, levels of nitrogen compounds are building up in soil, in the atmosphere and in water.

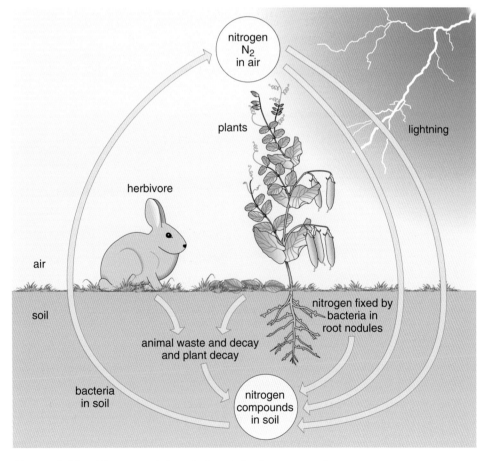

**Figure 3.20** The natural (pre-industrial) nitrogen cycle.

## Effects on humans

The most well-known effect of nitrates on human health is methaemoglobinaemia (met-heem-oh-gloh-bin-eem-ia) or 'blue baby syndrome'. If large quantities of nitrogen compounds are ingested in drinking water, the ability of the blood to carry oxygen is impaired, causing headache, fatigue, breathing difficulties, diarrhoea and vomiting and, in extreme cases, loss of consciousness and death. This syndrome is quite common in parts of the USA, and the Netherlands, where nitrogen levels are very high. Safety levels for nitrogen compounds in drinking water are set with a view to preventing methaemoglobinaemia in infants, an acute condition, and do not take into account the possible chronic health effects, for adults as well as children, of ingesting nitrogen compounds at low levels over a long period.

The oxygen-carrying capacity of the blood, and the symptoms that occur when oxygen levels are low are discussed in another book in this series (Midgley, 2008).

Nitrogen compounds are thought to be linked to asthma in some localities. Fresno, in the San Joaquin Valley of California is notorious for its smog and has the third highest asthma rate in the USA. Fresno is the centre of a major milk-producing region and dairy farms release large amounts of nitrogen in the form of ammonia which forms particulates in the air (Hooper, 2006). The increased use of nitrogen compounds in agriculture is also indirectly implicated in the marked increase in the incidence of asthma in many developed countries. Crops grown in nitrogen-enriched soils grow profusely and their flowers release very large amounts of pollen into the air (Townsend et al., 2003).

The most serious health consequences for humans from nitrogen pollution may well arise indirectly through its effects on the environment. For example, high levels of nitrogen in water cause the formation of algal bloom (Figure 3.21), exceptional growths of plant-like organisms, called algae, often combined with bacteria, which 'choke' lakes, rivers and streams. These blooms may contain a

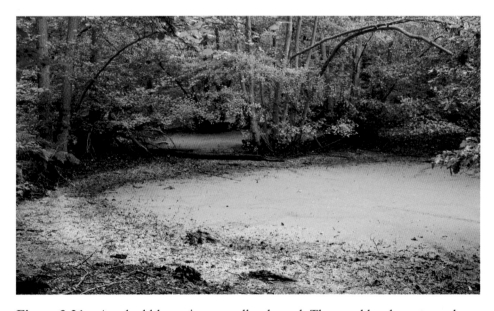

**Figure 3.21**   An algal bloom in a woodland pond. The pond has been turned green by the growth of algae, which covers the surface and prevents light and oxygen reaching plants and animals underneath. (Photo: Michaek Marten/Science Photo Library)

type of bacteria, called cyanobacteria, which produce toxins, killing water life and posing a threat to people. Algal blooms can kill the fish stocks on which many people may be dependent for food and it can take many years to clear them and restore the natural water ecology.

◆ From what you have read earlier, what other health threat arises when algal blooms form?

◆ As described in Section 3.4.2, algal blooms provide an ideal habitat for *V. cholerae*.

### 3.6.4 Endocrine disruptors

Then he was a she…

(Lou Reed, American rock singer)

In 1996, a book called *Our Stolen Future* was published, bringing to public attention a debate that had been simmering among biologists for some time. Written by Theo Colborn and two colleagues at the World Wildlife Fund (WWF), this book presented the hypothesis that certain industrial chemicals, commonly found as environmental pollutants, are threatening human health by disrupting the body's hormonal system. These chemicals, variously called **endocrine disruptors** (end-oh-krin), hormone mimics or, in the media, 'gender benders', could be playing a role in a range of problems, from reproductive and developmental abnormalities, to defects of the nervous system, to cancer. This disturbing hypothesis was based on studies of both wild and laboratory animals, for which there was a steady accumulation of evidence that certain xenobiotic chemicals were disrupting normal development and reproduction. One of the commonest examples of endocrine disruption involves, to varying extents, the feminisation of males. There seem to be no endocrine disruptors that masculinise females, but several disrupt the normal functioning of the female reproductive system (US Environmental Protection Agency, 1997).

While it is now widely accepted that endocrine disruptors are having serious effects on a variety of wild animals, there is considerable debate among biologists as to whether human health and reproduction are being affected. If it is, it represents a possible cost of living in the modern 'human zoo'.

Endocrine disruptors get their name because they interact with the endocrine (hormonal) system in the body. The **endocrine system** consists primarily of a number of endocrine glands (also known as ductless glands) that each secrete one or more hormones directly into the bloodstream. A **hormone** is a substance produced by an endocrine gland that is carried by the bloodstream to other organs or tissues where it acts to alter their structure or function.

An important effect of some hormones is to regulate behaviour. This is true of the 'flight or fight' hormone epinephrine (formerly known as adrenalin) which, secreted by the suprarenal glands in response to danger and other alarming stimuli, activates the body and facilitates a rapid response (Section 1.5). It is less true of sex hormones, such as oestrogen or testosterone, which have little immediate effect on behaviour, but which have a profound, long-term, *organising* effect on the body. Thus, the level of testosterone determines the timing of adolescence in boys, for example. This organising effect is important in the context of endocrine disruption because it means that, if an organism's endocrine system is disrupted early in life, it can have profound consequences that can affect it throughout its life.

Fundamental to understanding how hormones and endocrine disruptors work is the concept of a receptor. A **receptor** is a large, specialised molecular structure embedded in the membrane that forms the outer layer of a cell (Figure 3.22). It consists primarily of proteins that have affinity for a specific hormone, drug or other natural or synthetic chemical. For example, cells in the mammary glands of mammals have receptors on their surface with a special affinity for the hormone oestrogen, which is secreted primarily by the ovaries. When oestrogen comes into contact with an oestrogen receptor on a cell, it initiates a change within that cell. By this mechanism, oestrogen controls mammary development at adolescence and function during reproduction. Mammary glands are said to be 'target organs' of oestrogen. This 'special affinity' involves a process called binding, in which a specific part of a hormone molecule becomes attached to part of the corresponding receptor on the surface of the target cell, triggering a change within the target cell. You will see animations that illustrate this in Activity 3.2 on the DVD associated with this book. Because of the specificity of this relationship, the process of binding is often likened to a key being inserted into a lock (Figure 3.22).

Endocrine disruptors work because, although they are not hormones, and often bear no obvious similarity to hormones, they happen to have in their molecular structure, features that mimic the 'key' section of specific hormone molecules. Thus a substance that is not a hormone has the ability to 'unlock the lock' on target organs, which then behave as if the relevant hormone had become bound to them.

Before going on to examine endocrine disruptors in more detail, it is important to mention a related issue, the presence in the environment of real hormones. Women taking the contraceptive pill excrete substantial amounts of modified

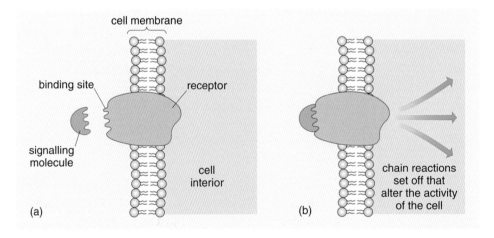

**Figure 3.22**  The 'lock and key' interaction between a signalling molecule (e.g. a hormone) and its specific receptor.

versions of human reproductive hormones, such as oestrogen, in their urine. Artificial hormones are not broken down in sewage treatment plants and so appear, sometimes in quite high concentrations, in sewage outflows into rivers. At a number of sites in the UK, male fish have been found to be feminised close to sewage outflows (Tyler et al., 1998). Now turn to Activity 3.2.

## Activity 3.2  Oestrogen mimics

Allow 45 minutes for this activity.

Now would be the ideal time to study the DVD activity entitled 'Oestrogen mimics' which you will find on the DVD associated with this book. The purpose of this activity is help you understand how certain manufactured chemicals in the environment disrupt the endocrine hormone system of humans and other animals, taking compounds called alkylphenols as the example.

The activity starts with a molecular model of the oestrogen receptor with a form of oestrogen called oestradiol present in the active site. Then, using a schematic model of the active site and molecular models of a range of compounds with varying activities as oestrogen mimics, you will be given the opportunity to discover interactively some of the molecular features that predispose a substance to act as an endocrine disruptor.

After completing this activity, you should have a better understating of why certain substances are oestrogen mimics, and why some are more potent than others.

If you are unable to play this sequence now, try to do so as soon as possible. You will find it harder to study the rest of this chapter until you have done so.

One of the molecular features – **hydroxyl groups** – are involved in the formation of hydrogen bonds, which were described in DVD Activity 3.1.

It is important to emphasise that animals are very sensitive to very small variations in reproductive hormones. This is illustrated by work carried out by an American biologist, Fred vom Saal, who works on rodents (vom Saal and Bronson, 1978, vom Saal et al., 1999). Rodents have large litters and, during their development within their mother, embryos are lined up in the uterus in a row. In this row a male embryo may find itself between another two males, between two females, or between one of each. Vom Saal developed techniques to determine the exact position of each embryo prior to birth and to detect small variations in the behaviour of the young rodents that those embryos became as they grew up. He found that the behaviour of individuals was affected by their position in the uterus, as measured by variations in aggressive and sexual behaviour. Male rodents that had been between another two males in the uterus are more aggressive and sexually active than those that had been between two females. This effect is due to the fact that, even as embryos, young mammals secrete tiny quantities of sex hormones. This example gives credence to the hypothesis that very small amounts of hormone, or of hormone mimics, can influence animals as they develop.

### The evidence for endocrine disruption in wildlife

During the 1970s and 1980s, biologists found alligators in Florida with reduced penis size and low fertility. About the same time Western gulls in the USA were found with abnormal mating behaviour and reproductive organs. These anomalies were linked to high levels of PCBs (polychlorinated biphenyls), DDT and dioxin in the local environment. Around the same time, reproductive abnormalities were found in fish living in British rivers close to sewage outfalls. Such findings stimulated ecotoxicologists to start looking closely at a range of xenobiotic chemicals and their possible endocrine-disrupting effects.

For example, atrazine is the most widely used herbicide in the world; 30 000 tons of it are sprayed onto farmland in the USA each year. It can be detected at quite high levels in streams and rivers that collect run-off from farmland and has been detected at high levels in rain. In a laboratory study, tadpoles of the African clawed frog (*Xenopus laevis*) were reared in water containing atrazine at concentrations similar to those found in natural water bodies in the USA. The tadpoles grew, developed and metamorphosed into frogs, at which point they were examined in detail. Many of them were hermaphrodites, meaning that their gonads (testes and ovaries) contained both egg- and sperm-producing tissues. Many of those that were unequivocally male had a poorly developed larynx, the means by which males produce mating calls. Males that were allowed to develop to adult age showed a ten-fold decrease in testosterone level compared with untreated males (Hayes et al., 2002a, b).

### The evidence for endocrine disruption in humans

Establishing a link between endocrine disruptors and human health is complicated by the fact that experiments of the kind conducted on animals are out of the question. It would be wholly unethical to administer DDT to people, for example, to see what effects it had on them. Studies on humans are thus limited to establishing a correlation between the presence of a xenobiotic chemical in the environment and some kind of health problem.

For example, the Aamjiwnaang are a community of Native Americans who live next to a major chemical complex in Ontario, Canada. Over the years, the ratio of boys and girls born in this community has been changing, from equal numbers in the period 1984–88 to 46 boys and 86 girls in 1999–2003. High levels of phthalates and hexachlorobenzene, both known to have endocrine-disrupting properties, have been found in the local soil (Mackenzie et al., 2005). Such data are suggestive of a causal link between endocrine-disrupting chemicals and a changed sex ratio, but do not provide conclusive proof for such a link. There may be other reasons why the sex ratio has changed.

By 2006, over 50 chemical compounds had been identified as endocrine disruptors. Many of these are long-lived compounds that can persist in the environment for many years without being degraded, and which can bioaccumulate in body tissues. They include several herbicides (e.g. atrazine), fungicides, and insecticides (e.g. DDT); industrial chemicals and by-products such as PCBs and dioxin; and a number of compounds found in plastics, such as phthalates and styrenes, that are used to package foods and drinks (WRI, 1999). Levels of endocrine disruptors are especially high in heavily urbanised areas of the world.

### 3.6.5 Postscript to Section 3.6

This section has considered a small number of chemical pollutants of water and has examined what is known about their harmful effects on animals, humans and the environment. You should be aware of a number of important general points that arise from what you have read. First, there is an enormous variety of chemical pollutants; you have read about only a few. Secondly, the evidence that chemical pollutants are potentially harmful is often more convincing from studies of animals than it is from studies of human health. Thirdly, you have read mostly about amphibians; much is known about the harmful effects of chemical pollutants on other animals, but they have been the focus here because of their role as 'canaries', possibly providing early warning of environmental problems (Chapter 1). Finally, while much is known about the harmful effects of chemical pollutants on wildlife and people, this body of knowledge pales into insignificance in comparison with what is not known.

## 3.7 Postscript to this book

Water is a natural resource that is vital to human health. It is also a resource that is undergoing a major crisis; its capacity to support plant and animal life is rapidly being destroyed by human activities. The message of this book is that human health and the health of the natural environment are intimately linked to one another.

> 'Perhaps the time has come to cease calling it the "environmentalist view", as though it were a lobbying effort outside the mainstream of human activity, and start calling it the real-world view'.
>
> E. O. Wilson (American biologist and environmental campaigner)

## Summary of Chapter 3

3.1 Freshwater is a finite and limited resource on Earth and, increasingly, much of it is polluted, by both pathogenic microbes and chemical contaminants.

3.2 Human demand for freshwater is increasing; in particular, water is required to irrigate crops to feed the rapidly expanding human population.

3.3 Water cycles globally, through the oceans, the atmosphere and freshwater river systems. At certain points in the cycle, water is purified, both naturally and by treatment plants.

3.4 Freshwater is very unevenly distributed in the world, such that a large proportion of the world's human population has insufficient water for growing crops, for drinking and for sanitation.

3.5 Water is a chemical compound made of molecules, each of which is composed of two hydrogen atoms attached to an oxygen atom. Water molecules are extremely small (of the order $10^{-10}$ m across) and so models are used to visualise their behaviour.

3.6 Water is a very good solvent. This stems from the fact that it is a polar molecule, with negatively- and positively-charged regions, and can form hydrogen bonds. As a consequence it can dissolve both ionic compounds such as sodium chloride and molecular compounds such as amino acids or sugars made up of polar molecules.

3.7 Climate change is altering the global distribution of water, causing droughts in some regions, flooding in others.

3.8 The chemical and physical properties of water are such that, over the range of temperatures that occur on Earth, it supports a rich diversity of plants and animals.

3.9 Water-borne infectious diseases threaten human health wherever water supplies are contaminated by pathogenic microbes, and where there is inadequate sanitation.

3.10 Diarrhoeal diseases are caused by a variety of water-borne pathogens, including *Vibrio cholerae* (cholera) and *Cryptosporidium* (cryptosporidiosis).

3.11 Diarrhoeal diseases cause a vicious circle of water-loss and malnutrition that, in children, stunts growth and development, causes immunodeficiency, and increases susceptibility to other infectious diseases.

3.12 The control of cholera is complicated by the fact that its pathogen, *V. cholerae*, is a free-living organism, living in both freshwater and marine habitats.

3.13 The chemical pollution of freshwater and coastal habitats favours the proliferation of algae that harbour *V. cholerae*, increasing the risk of cholera.

3.14 Diarrhoeal diseases can be treated by 'point-of-use' strategies (i.e. close to where people live), such as filtering water and disinfection.

3.15 An enormous variety of chemical compounds, produced by human activities, pollute natural water bodies, causing both acute and chronic pollution.

3.16 Evidence for the effect of chemical pollution is provided by ecotoxicology, the study of the impact of xenobiotic chemicals on wildlife in natural situations.

3.17 As chemical pollutants pass through natural food chains, bioaccumulation causes high levels to build up at certain points, e.g. in the fat reserves of predatory fish and birds. As a result, these animals, and their offspring, can be exposed to a very high dose.

3.18 DDT is an effective insecticide that is toxic to wildlife, but is also a vital means for combating malaria.

3.19 Levels of mercury compounds in the environment are increasing; they are a threat to wildlife and to people who eat a lot of fish, and especially to their children.

3.20 Levels of nitrogen compounds in the environment are increasing very rapidly. These are toxic to humans at high levels but, more importantly, at lower levels they cause widespread environmental changes, especially eutrophication of water.

3.21 A large number of xenobiotic chemicals, called endocrine disruptors, cause major disruption to the reproductive development of freshwater animals; their possible effects on humans are uncertain.

## Learning outcomes for Chapter 3

After studying this chapter and its associated activities, you should be able to:

LO 3.1　Define and use in context, or recognise definitions and applications of, each of the terms printed in **bold** in the text (Questions 3.5 and 3.7 and DVD Activity 3.1)

LO 3.2　Identify some of the reasons why clean, freshwater is an increasingly scarce resource for many people in the world. (Question 3.1)

LO 3.3　Describe the structure of atoms in terms of a positively charged nucleus surrounded by negatively charged electrons. (DVD Activity 3.1)

LO 3.4　Describe how molecules are formed from atoms joined together by chemical bonds. (DVD Activity 3.1)

LO 3.5　Describe the structure, size, shape, and electron distribution of the water molecule, including the formation of hydrogen bonds, and explain its ability to act as a solvent in terms of these properties. (DVD Activity 3.1)

LO 3.6　Describe the process by which sodium chloride dissolves in water and recognise that many common substances present in mineral water (e.g. sulfates and nitrates) are polyatomic ions. (DVD Activity 3.1)

LO 3.7　Describe the 'vicious cycle' that links diarrhoeal diseases to nutrition, stature and infectious diseases. (Question 3.2)

LO 3.8　Discuss aspects of the biology of *Vibrio cholerae* that have implications for the way attempts are made to control cholera. (Question 3.3)

LO 3.9　Describe examples of 'point-of-use' strategies to combat water-borne infections. (Question 3.4 and DVD Activity 3.1)

LO 3.10　Explain what is meant by the bioaccumulation of xenobiotic chemicals and identify the implications that this has for what people can safely eat. (Question 3.5)

LO 3.11　Distinguish between the effects on human health of high and low levels of environmental pollution by nitrogen compounds. (Question 3.6)

LO 3.12　Explain what is meant by an endocrine disruptor. (Question 3.7 and DVD Activity 3.2)

LO 3.13　Recognise the presence of certain groups of atoms in a molecule (e.g. hydroxyl groups) that increase the probability of that compound being an endocrine disruptor. (DVD Activity 3.2)

If you are studying this book as part of an Open University course, you should also be able to:

LO 3.14  Conduct a guided internet search to retrieve, record and tabulate international data on mortality from diarrhoeal diseases and access to clean water and improved sanitation. (Activity C3 in the *Companion*)

## Self-assessment questions for Chapter 3

You had the opportunity to demonstrate LOs 3.3 to 3.6 and 3.13 by answering questions in DVD Activities 3.1 and 3.2.

### Question 3.1 (LO 3.2)

Give three reasons why many people in the world face an increasingly severe shortage of fresh, safe water.

### Question 3.2 (LO 3.7)

Why are nutritional deficiencies and infectious diseases regarded as linked medical problems?

### Question 3.3 (LO 3.8)

Why is the control of cholera made difficult by the fact that (a) cholera has a high infectious dose and, (b) that *Vibrio cholerae* lives naturally in aquatic habitats?

### Question 3.4 (LO 3.9)

Give two examples of 'point-of-use' strategies used to combat water-borne infections in drinking water.

### Question 3.5 (LOs 3.1 and 3.10)

In some parts of the world, people are advised to limit the amount of certain kinds of fish that they eat; why is this?

### Question 3.6 (LO 3.11)

Describe how, as levels of nitrogen compounds increase in the environment, their effects on human health change.

### Question 3.7 (LOs 3.1 and 3.12)

What does it mean to say that a particular xenobiotic chemical is an endocrine disruptor?

# ANSWERS TO SELF-ASSESSMENT QUESTIONS

## Question 1.1

The female pelvis is wider than the optimum for running quickly to allow space for the relatively large brain of a human baby to pass through during childbirth. Babies are born long before their brains reach adult size. This increases their mother's survival chances because she can have a more compact pelvis than would otherwise be required, which in turn enables her to run faster in escaping from predators.

## Question 1.2

Coal miners used to take canaries underground because they were more sensitive than humans to the toxic effects of dangerous gases building up in the mine. The alarming increase in the rate of extinction of amphibians has led some biologists to liken them to canaries in the coal mine, because they may be more sensitive than other species to the pollutants arising from human settlements, vehicles and industrial processes.

## Question 1.3

The SARS epidemic threatened to become a pandemic because it was transported very rapidly between continents by air travellers who had been in contact with an infected person. This illustrates the speed with which infectious disease can spread among the highly mobile population of the modern world.

## Question 1.4

The World Bank classification is based solely on national income, but the WHO also takes into account certain development indicators such as access to education, health care, sanitation and clean water when deciding whether a country is 'developed' or 'developing'. The discrepancy between the World Bank and WHO classifications of Singapore suggest that, despite its high income, the health and other development indicators of *most* people in Singapore were below the standard of other wealthy nations. This illustrates that inequalities in the *distribution* of wealth within a population can have a major impact on the health of its people.

## Question 1.5

The percentage of obese children in at least one of the age-groups is always greater than in the immediately preceding period. In the 1960s and early 1970s, there was a higher proportion of obese teenagers than among the 6- to 11-year-olds, but as time passed the younger ones caught up. In 1999–2002, 16% of children in both age-groups were obese, roughly three times the proportion up to 1980.

The most likely explanation for this trend is that American children in this period were eating more and exercising less; the gap between their energy in-take and the energy they expended appears to have got larger over time, so that more of them stored the food they consumed as fat.

## Question 1.6

Figure 1.27 shows that blood pressure increases with age after 40 years even in people in a relatively low-stress working environment. Therefore, if you did not take account of the age of the subjects in your study, you might wrongly attribute cases of high blood pressure to whatever stressor was being investigated. In reality high blood pressure may simply have been due to normal age-related increases.

## Question 2.1

Tetanus was the 18th most common cause of death in 1990, but had fallen off the bottom of the table by 2002. (You may be interested to know that the improvement is mainly due to the widespread anti-tetanus vaccination of children in developing countries, who are most at risk from this infection.)

## Question 2.2

The proportion of all DALYs in Tanzania in 2002 which were attributable to road traffic accidents was:

$$\frac{374\,000}{20\,240\,000} \times 100 = 1.8\%,$$

compared with 1.4% in the UK.

## Question 2.3

Figure 2.7 shows that the distribution of deaths *and* DALYs attributable to alcohol disproportionately affects people aged 15–59 years. 65% of all deaths due to alcohol and 87% of all DALYs due to alcohol occur in this age-group.

## Question 2.4

(a) Risk factors associated with infectious and parasitic diseases in developing countries: unsafe sex, unsafe water supply and poor sanitation. You may also have suggested underweight as an indirect risk factor for these diseases because it increases susceptibility to infection.

(b) Risk factors associated with chronic non-communicable diseases in developing countries: tobacco and alcohol consumption, urban air pollution, indoor air pollution from cooking fires, overweight and obesity, underweight and iron-deficiency anaemia.

(c) Unsafe water supply, poor sanitation and indoor air pollution from cooking fires are not significant causes of disease in developed countries.

## Question 2.5

In powers of ten notation, 0.3 μm would be written as $3 \cdot 10^{-7}$ m (three times ten to the minus seven metres). This is the same as $0.3 \times 10^{-6}$ m, but the convention in science is that the multiplier must always be a number between 1 and 10. The power is negative ($10^{-7}$) because the length of this bacterium is *less* than 1 metre (much less!).

## Question 3.1

The human population of the world is increasing rapidly; per capita use of freshwater is increasing; climate change is altering the distribution of freshwater, making it more scarce in some regions, such as southern Africa. You might also have answered, correctly, that an increasing proportion of water supplies are polluted, by pathogens and by xenobiotic chemicals, as a result of increasing urbanisation and industrialisation.

## Question 3.2

They are linked because they form part of a 'vicious cycle' that involves a reduction in the efficiency of the immune system. Malnutrition leads to immunodeficiency which reduces the body's capacity to resist infectious diseases. Infectious diseases, particularly those affecting the gut (e.g. cholera), prevent the intake of adequate nutrition.

## Question 3.3

(a) Individuals can be infected by low doses of *V. cholerae* and even though they themselves may not become ill, they can still spread the disease.

(b) A pathogenic microbe that lives only in people can, at least potentially, be controlled by vaccinating people and getting them to change their behaviour. Such measures have no impact on *V. cholerae* living in natural water bodies.

## Question 3.4

Disinfectants can be added to drinking water to lower the level of pathogenic microbes. Filtering drinking water through sari cloth removes the microscopic plankton that harbour *V. cholerae*, the pathogen that causes cholera.

## Question 3.5

Large, predatory fish occupy a position at the top of food chains in which, by bioaccumulation, they can contain high levels of xenobiotic chemicals, such as methyl mercury, which may be harmful to health, particularly during fetal development.

## Question 3.6

At lower levels, nitrogen compounds cause deterioration, by eutrophication, of natural water bodies, which can promote the formation of algal blooms. This can have indirect effects on human health, by depleting fish stocks on which some communities depend. At higher levels, they can have a direct impact on human health, for example, by causing 'blue baby' syndrome, and also asthma in some localities.

## Question 3.7

An endocrine disruptor is a chemical compound which, though not itself a hormone, has a molecular structure that enables it to mimic the effect of a hormone in an animal. The commonest examples of endocrine disruptors are those that mimic female hormones and feminise male animals (e.g. fish).

# REFERENCES AND FURTHER READING

## References

Altmann, P., Cunningham, J., Dhanesha, U., Ballard, M., Thompson, J. and Marsh, F. (1999) 'Disturbance of cerebral function in people exposed to drinking water contaminated with aluminium sulphate: retrospective study of the Camelford water incident', *British Medical Journal*, vol. 319, pp. 807–811.

AmphibiaWeb (2007) [online]. Available from: http://elib.cs.berkeley.edu/aw/ (Accessed March 2007)

Bank, M. S., Crocker, J. B., Davis, S., Brotherton, D. K., Cook, R., Behler, J. and Connery, B. (2006) 'Population decline of northern dusky salamanders at Acadia National Park, Maine, USA', *Biological Conservation*, vol. 130, pp. 230–238.

Beard, J. (2006) 'DDT and human health', *Science of the Total Environment*, vol. 355, pp. 78–89.

Boening, D. W. (2000) 'Ecological effects, transport, and fate of mercury: a general review', *Chemosphere*, vol. 40, pp. 1335–1351.

Booth, S. and Zeller, D. (2005) 'Mercury, food webs, and marine mammals: implications of diet and climate change for human health', *Environmental Health Perspectives*, vol. 113, pp. 521–526.

Brown, P. (2002) Fish clue to human fertility decline, *Guardian*, 18 March 2002, p. 9.

Bumb, B and Baanante, C. (1996) *World Trends in Fertilizer Use and Projections to 2020*, Brief No. 38, International Food Policy Research Institute, Washington, D.C.

Cancer Research UK (2007) [online]. Available from: http://www.cancerhelp. org.uk/help/default.asp?page=3005 (Accessed March 2007)

Carlson, N. R. (2001) *Physiology of Behavior* (7th edn), Boston, Allyn & Bacon.

Clean Air Network (1999) *Mercury sources factsheet* [online]. Available from: www.cleanair.net (Accessed March 2006)

Cliff, A. and Haggett, P. (2004) 'Time, travel and infection', *British Medical Bulletin*, vol. 69, pp. 87–99.

Cohen, J. T., Bellinger, D. C. and Shaywitz, B. A. (2005) 'A quantitative analysis of prenatal methyl mercury exposure and cognitive development', *American Journal of Preventive Medicine*, vol. 29, pp. 353–365.

Colborn, T., Dumanoski, D. and Myers, J. P. (1996) *Our Stolen Future*, Abacus.

Colwell, R. R. et al. (2003) 'Reduction of cholera in Bangladeshi villages by simple filtration', *Proceedings of the National Academy of Sciences USA*, vol. 100, pp. 1051–1055.

Connell, D., Lam, P., Richardson, B. and Wu, R. (1999) *Introduction to Ecotoxicology*, Oxford, Blackwell Science.

Cottingham, K. L., Chiavelli, D. A. and Taylor, R. K. (2003) 'Environmental microbe and human pathogen: the ecology and microbiology of *Vibrio cholera*', *Frontiers in Ecology and the Environment*, vol. 1, pp. 870–86.

Dobzhansky, T. (1973) 'Nothing in biology makes sense except in the light of evolution', *The American Biology Teacher*, vol. 35, pp. 125–129.

Dunbar, R. (1991) 'Foraging for nature's balanced diet', *New Scientist,* 3 August 1991, pp. 25–28.

Dunbar, R. (2004) *The Human Story. A New History of Mankind's Evolution*, London, Faber & Faber.

Dunbar, R. and Barrett, L. (2000) *Cousins*, BBC Worldwide.

Epstein, P. R. (2005) 'Climate change and human health', *New England Journal of Medicine*, vol. 353, pp. 1433–1436.

Epstein, P. R., Ford, T. E. and Colwell, R. R. (1993) 'Health and climate change: marine ecosystems', *The Lancet*, vol. 342, pp. 1216–1219.

Foley, J. A. et al. (2005) 'Global consequences of land use', *Science*, vol. 309, pp. 570–574.

Freedman, B. (1989) *Environmental Ecology* (2nd edn), San Diego, Academic Press.

Furlow, B. (2005) 'To your good health!' *New Scientist*, 3 December 2005, pp. 47–49.

Galloway, J. N., Aber, J. D., Erisman, J. W., Seitzinger, S. P., Howarth, R. W., Cowling, E. B. and Cosby, B. J. (2003) 'The nitrogen cascade', *BioScience,* vol. 53, pp. 341–356.

GACVS (2006) [online] *Statement on thiomersal*, Global Advisory Committee on Vaccine Safety, Geneva, World Health Organization. Available from: http://www.who.int/vaccine_safety/topics/thiomersal/statement200308/en/index.html (Accessed 20 February 2007)

Gedney, N., Cox, P. M., Betts, R. A., Boucher, O., Huntingford, C. and Stott, P. A. (2006) 'Detection of a direct carbon dioxide effect in continental river runoff records', *Nature*, vol. 439, pp. 835–838.

Gillespie, S. and Bamford, K. (2000) *Medical Microbiology and Infection at a Glance*, Oxford, Blackwell Science.

Gleick, P. H. (2003) 'Water use', *Annual Review of Environment and Resources*, vol. 28, pp. 275–314.

Global Amphibian Assessment (2007) [online]. Available from: www.globalamphibians.org (Accessed March 2007)

Griffiths, R. A., de Wijer, P. and May, R. T. (1994) 'The effect of pH on the development of eggs and larvae of smooth and palmate newts, *Triturus vulgaris* and *T. helveticus*', *Journal of Zoology*, vol. 230, pp. 401–409.

Halliday, T. (2000) 'Do frogs make good canaries?' *The Biologist*, vol. 47, pp. 143–146.

Haslam, D. W. and James, W. P. T. (2005) 'Obesity', *The Lancet*, vol. 366, pp. 1197–1209.

Hayes, T. B. et al. (2002a) 'Hermaphroditic, demasculinized frogs after exposure to the herbicide atrazine at low ecologically relevant doses', *Proceedings of the National Academy of Sciences USA*, vol. 99, pp. 5476–5480.

Hayes, T. B. et al. (2002b) 'Feminization of male frogs in the wild', *Nature*, vol. 419, pp. 895–896.

Hecht, J. (2006) 'Losing the ground beneath their feet', *New Scientist*, 18 February 2006, pp. 8–9.

Hightower, J. M., O'Hare, A. and Hernandez, G. T. (2006) 'Blood mercury reporting in NHANES: identifying Asian, Pacific Islander, Native American, and multiracial groups', *Environmental Health Perspectives*, vol. 114, pp. 173–175.

Hooper, R. (2006) 'Something in the air', *New Scientist*, 21 January 2006, pp. 40–43.

Houghton, J. (2004) *Global Warming. The Complete Briefing* (3rd edn), Cambridge, Cambridge University Press.

IPCC (2007) *Climate Change 2007: The Physical Science Basis. Contribution of Working group I to the Fourth Assessment Report of the Intergovernmental Panel on Climate Change*, Cambridge University Press. 'Summary for Policymakers' [online]. Available from: www.ipcc.ch/ (Accessed 20 February 2007)

Jung, R. T. (1997) 'Obesity as a disease', *British Medical Journal*, vol. 53, pp. 307–321.

Kalkstein, L. S. and Smoyer, K. E. (1993) 'The impact of climate change on human health: some international implications', *Cellular and Molecular Life Sciences*, vol. 49, pp. 969–979.

King's Fund (2006) Briefing: Local variations in NHS spending priorities [online] Available from: www.kingsfund.org.uk (Accessed February 2007)

Kosek, M., Bern, C. and Guerrant, R. L. (2003) 'The global burden of diarrhoeal disease, as estimated from studies published between 1992 and 2000', *Bulletin of the WHO*, vol. 81, pp. 197–204.

Lake, I. R., Bentham, G., Kovatys, R. S. and Nichols, G. L. (2005) 'Effects of weather and river flow on cryptosporidiosis', *Journal of Water Health*, vol. 3, pp. 469–474.

Lannoo, M., Funk, C., Gadd, M., Halliday, T. and Mitchell, J. (2007) 'Freshwater resources and associated terrestrial landscapes', in Gascon, C., Collins, J. P., Moore, R. D., Church, D. R., McKay, J. and Mendelson III, J. R. (eds) *Amphibian Conservation Action Plan*, IUCN, Gland, Switzerland and Cambridge, UK, IUCN/SSC Amphibian Specialist Group.

Lee, S. H., Levy, D. A., Craun, G. F., Beach, M. J. and Caldreon, R. L. (2002) 'Surveillance for waterborne-disease outbreaks - United States, 1999-2000', *Morbidity and Mortality Weekly Report Surveillance Summaries*, vol. 51, pp.1–47.

Lewin, R. (1999) *Human Evolution* (4th edn), Oxford, Blackwell Science.

Linder, G. and Grillitsch, B. (2000) 'Ecotoxicology of metals', in Sparling, D. W., Linder, G. and Bishop C. A. (eds) *Ecotoxicology of Amphibians and Reptiles*,' SETAC Press, pp. 325–459.

Lougheed, T. (2006) 'A clear solution for dirty water', *Environmental Health Perspectives*, vol. 114, A424–A427.

Lucas, R. M., McMichael, T., Smith, W. and Armstrong, B. (2006) Solar ultraviolet radiation. Global burden of disease due to ultraviolet radiation', *Environmental Burden of Disease Series*, No. 13, Geneva, World Health Organization.

Mackenzie, C. A., Lockridge, A and Keith, M. (2005) 'Declining sex ratio in a First Nation community', *Environmental Health Perspectives*, vol. 113, pp. 1295–1298.

MacKenzie, W. R. et al. (1994) 'A massive outbreak in Milwaukee of cryptosporidium infection transmitted through the public water supply', *New England Journal of Medicine*, vol. 331, pp. 161–167.

McEvedy, C. and Jones, R. (1978) *Atlas of World Population*, New York, Viking.

McLannahan, H. (ed.) (2008) *Visual Impairment: A Global View*, Oxford, Oxford University Press, in press.

Maddison, A. (2001) *The World Economy: a Millennial Perspective.* Organisation for Economic Cooperation and Development (OECD)

Marshall, J. (2005) 'Megacity, mega mess', *Nature*, vol. 437, pp. 312–314.

Matthews, D. (2006) 'The water cycle freshens up', *Nature*, vol. 439, pp. 793–794.

Meinhardt, P. L., Casemore, D. P. and Miller, K. B. (1996) 'Epidemiologic aspects of human cryptosporidiosis and the role of waterborne transmission', *Epidemiologic Reviews*, vol. 18, pp. 118–136.

Melzer, D. et al. (2002) The social and economic circumstances of adults with mental disorders, London, HMSO.

Midgley, C. A. (ed.) (2008) *Chronic Obstructive Pulmonary Disease: A Forgotten Killer*, Oxford, Oxford University Press, in press.

Monteiro, C. A., Moura, E. C., Conde, W. L. and Popkin, B. M. (2004) 'Socioeconomic status and obesity in adult populations of developing countries: a review', *Bulletin of the WHO*, vol. 82, pp. 940–946.

Morris, D. (1969) *The Human Zoo*, London, Jonathan Cape.

Murray, C. J. L. and Lopez, A. D. (1997a) 'Global mortality disability, and the contribution of risk factors: Global Burden of Disease study', *The Lancet*, vol. 349, pp. 1436–1442.

Murray, C. J. L. and Lopez, A. D. (1997b) 'Mortality by cause for eight regions of the world: Global Burden of Disease study', *The Lancet*, vol. 349, pp. 1269–1276.

Nestle, M. (2006) 'Food marketing and childhood obesity – a matter of policy', *New England Journal of Medicine*, vol. 354, pp. 2527–2529.

OECD (2005) *Health at a Glance. OECD Indicators 2005.* Organisation for Economic Co-operation and Development.

Parvin, E. M. (ed.) (2007) *Screening for Breast Cancer*, Oxford, Oxford University Press, in press.

Patz, J. A. and Kovats, R. S. (2002) 'Hotspots in climate change and human health', *British Medical Journal*, vol. 325, pp. 1094–1098.

Patz, J. A., Campbell-Lendrum, D., Holloway, T. and Foley, J. A. (2005) 'Impact of regional climate change on human health', *Nature*, vol. 438, pp. 310–317.

Phillips, J. B. (ed.) (2008) *Trauma, Repair and Recovery*, Oxford, Oxford University Press, in press.

Pimm, S. L., Russell, G. J., Gittleman, J. L. and Brooks, T. M. (1995) 'The future of biodiversity', *Science*, vol. 269, pp. 347–350.

Porter, R. (1997) *The Greatest Benefit to Mankind*, London, Harper Collins.

Rahman, A., Lee, H. K. and Khan, M. A. (1997) 'Domestic water contamination in rapidly growing megacities of Asia: case of Karachi, Pakistan', *Environmental Monitoring and Assessment*, vol. 44, pp. 339–360.

Rodgers, A., Ezzati, M., Vander Hoorn, S., Lopez, A. D., Lin, R-B. and Murray, C. J. L. (2004) 'Distribution of major health risks: findings from the global burden of disease study', *PLoS Medicine*, vol. 1, pp. 44–55.

Sargent, M. G. (2005) *Biomedicine and the Human Condition*, Cambridge University Press.

Schiermeier, Q. (2005) 'The chaos to come', *Nature*, vol. 438, pp. 903–906.

Schweiger, L. (2005) 'Keeping tabs on mercury', *The Scientist*, 24 October 2005, pp. 10.

Scrimshaw, N. S. (2003) 'Historical concepts of interactions, synergism and antagonism between nutrition and infection', *Journal of Nutrition*, vol. 133, pp. 316S–321S.

Smart, L.E. (ed.) (2007) *Alcohol and Human Health*, Oxford, Oxford University Press, in press.

Tilman, D., Fargione, J., Wolff, B., D'Antonio, C., Dobson, A., Howarth, R., Schindler, D., Schlesinger, W. H., Simberloff, D. and Swackhamer, D. (2001) 'Forecasting agriculturally driven global environmental change', *Science*, vol. 292, pp. 281–284.

Toates, F. (2007) *Biological Psychology* (2nd edn), Harlow, Prentice Hall.

Townsend, A. R. et al. (2003) 'Human health effects of a changing global nitrogen cycle', *Frontiers in Ecology and the Environment*, vol. 1, pp. 240–246.

Tyler, C. R., Jobling, S. and Sumpter, J. P. (1998) 'Endocrine disruption in wildlife: a critical review of the evidence', *Critical Reviews in Toxicology*, vol. 28, pp. 319–361.

UK National Statistics (2007) [online]. Available from: www.statistics.gov.uk (Accessed March 2007)

UNESCO (2003) *Water for People, Water for Life*. The United Nations World Water Development Report. Available from: www.unesco.org/water/wwap (Accessed March 2007)

United Nations (2003) [online] *World Economic and Social Survey 2003*. Available from http://www.who.int/immunization_monitoring/glossary/en/index2.html (Accessed March 2007)

UN Millennium Development Goals (2005) [online]. Available from www.un.org/millenniumgoals (Accessed March 2007)

US Environmental Protection Agency (1997) *Special Report on Environmental Endocrine Disruption: An effects assessment and analysis*, Risk Assessment Forum report EPA/6.30/R-96/012, Washington D.C.

vom Saal, F. and Bronson, F. (1978) 'In utero proximity of female mouse fetuses to males: effect on reproductive performance during later life', *Biology of Reproduction*, vol. 19, pp. 842–853.

vom Saal, F. S., Clark, M. M., Galef, B. G., Drickamer, L. C. and Vandenbergh, J. G. (1999) 'The intrauterine position (IUP) phenomenon', in Knobil, E. and Neill, J. (eds) *Encyclopedia of Reproduction*, New York, Academic Press, Volume 2, pp. 893–900.

Watkins, K. (2006) *Beyond Scarcity: Power, Poverty and the Global Water Crisis.* Human Development Report 2006, United Nations Development Programme (UNDP).

WHO (2000) [online] Report on global surveillance of epidemic-prone infectious diseases – cholera. Geneva, World Health Organization. Available from: www.who.int/csr/resources/publications/cholera (Accessed March 2007)

WHO (2003) *World Health Annual Report, 2003*. Geneva, World Health Organization.

WHO (2004) *World Health Report 2004: Changing History*, Geneva, World Health Organization.

WHO (2005a) *World Health Report 2005: Make Every Mother and Child Count*, Geneva, World Health Organization.

WHO (2005b) *Mercury in Health Care.* (Policy Paper.)

WHO (2006) *World Health Statistics 2006*, Geneva, World Health Organization.

WHO (2007) [online] Depression. Available from: www.who.int/mental_health/management/depression/definition/en/ (Accessed 11 February 2007).

WRI (World Resources Institute) (1999) *World Resources 1998-99. A Guide to the Global Environment*, NewYork, Oxford University Press.

Wu, Y. (2006) 'Overweight and obesity in China', *British Medical Journal*, vol. 333, pp. 362–363.

Zahir, F., Rizwi, S. J., Haq, S. K. and Khan, R. H. (2005) 'Low dose mercury toxicity and human health', *Environmental Toxicology and Pharmacology*, vol. 20, pp. 351–360.

## Further reading

Clasen, T., Schmidt, W-P., Rabie, T., Roberts, I. and Cairncross, S. (2007) Interventions to improve water quality for preventing diarrhoea: systematic review and meta-analysis. *British Medical Journal*, vol. 334, p. 782.

OECD (2005) *Health at a Glance. OECD Indicators 2005*, Organisation for Economic Co-operation and Development.

Townsend, A. R. et al. (2003) 'Human health effects of a changing global nitrogen cycle', *Frontiers in Ecology and the Environment*, vol. 1, pp. 240–246.

WHO (2003) *World Health Report, 2003: Shaping the Future*, Geneva, World Health Organization.

WHO (2004) *World Health Report 2004: Changing History*, Geneva, World Health Organization.

WHO (2005) *World Health Report 2005: Make Every Mother and Child Count*, Geneva, World Health Organization.

WHO (2006) *World Health Statistics 2006*, Geneva, World Health Organization.

WRI (World Resources Institute) (1999) *World Resources 1998-99. A Guide to the Global Environment*, New York, Oxford University Press.

*Useful websites, maintained by the OU Library through the ROUTES system:*

http://www.who.int/healthinfo/en/ (WHO health information main page)

http://www.who.int/topics/en/   (WHO health topics A to Z)

http://www.who.int/healthinfo/bod/en/index.html (WHO Global Burden of Disease site)

http://www.who.int/water_sanitation_health/en/ (WHO water and sanitation site)

http://www.un.org/millenniumgoals/ (the UN millennium development goals 'home' site)

http://millenniumindicators.un.org/unsd/mdg/Default.aspx (UN database on progress towards achieving the millennium development goals)

http://www.wri.org/ (The World Resources Institute's 'home' site, providing access to a wide range of reports on natural resources, agriculture, climate change, human health, etc.)

# ACKNOWLEDGEMENTS

Grateful acknowledgement is made to the following sources for permission to reproduce material in this book.

*Figures*

Figure 1.1: Mark Edwards/Still Pictures; Figure 1.2: Jeremy Hartley/Panos Pictures; Figure 1.3 and 1.16a: Lewin, R. (1999) *Human Evolution* (4th edn), Blackwell Science; Figure 1.4: Yann Arthus-Bertrand/Impact Photos; Figure 1.5: Phillip Wolmuth/Panos Pictures; Figure 1.6: Shoeb Faruquie/DRIK; Figure 1.8: Images provided by Ozone Processing Team at NASA's Goddard Space Flight Center; Figure 1.10: www.who.int/immunization/glossary/en/index2.html. © Copyright World Health Organization (WHO), 2006. All rights reserved; Figure 1.11: Jeroen Daniel Kraan (Holland)/Flickr Photo Sharing; Figure 1.13: Marshall, J. (2005) 'Megacity, mega mess', *Nature*, vol. 437, Copyright © Nature Publishing Group; Figure 1.14: Tony Camacho/Science Photo Library; Figure 1.15: Caroline Pond; Figure 1.16b: Dr Franz B. M. de Waal, Living Links Center, Emory University; Figures 1.17, 1.18 and 1.20: *Health at a Glance – OECD Indicators 2005*, OECD Publishing; Figure 1.19: Mark Henley/Panos Pictures; Figure 1.21: Cliff, A. and Haggett, P. (2004) 'Time, travel and infection', *British Medical Bulletin*, vol. 69, The British Council; Figure 1.22: *WHO Report on Global Surveillance of Epidemic-Prone Infectious Diseases.* © Copyright World Health Organization (WHO). All rights reserved; Figure 1.23: www.who.int/whosis/whostat2006/en/index.html. © Copyright World Health Organization (WHO) 2006. All rights reserved; Figure 1.24: Wu, Y. (2006) 'Overweight and obesity in China', *British Medical Journal*, vol. 333, 19 Aug 2006. Copyright © 2006 BMJ Publishing Group Ltd; Figure 1.26: Kings Fund (2006) *Briefing: Local Variations in NHS Spending Priorities*, www.kingsfund.org.uk/resouces/briefings/figures/local_variations.html; Figure 1.27: Carson, N. R. (2001), *Physiology of Behaviour* (7th edn), Pearson Education Inc; Figure 1.28: Topham/EMPICS TopFoto.co.uk; Figure 1.29: Nestle, M. (2006) 'Food marketing and childhood obesity – a matter of policy', *New England Journal of Medicine*, vol. 354, p. 24, Massachusetts Medical Society;

Figure 2.1: Chris Sattiberger/Panos Pictures; Figure 2.3: Courtesy of the National Institute for Biological Standards and Control;

Figure 3.1: Global Environmental Teachings, University of Wisconsin: Stevens Point; Figures 3.3 and 3.5: Houghton, J. (2004) *Global Warming* (3rd edn), Cambridge University Press; Figure 3.7: Courtesy of Teaching Aids at Low Cost (TALC); Figure 3.8: Kosek, M., Bern, C. and Guerrant, R. L. (2003) 'The global burden of diarrhoeal disease as estimated from studies published between 1992 and 2000', *Bulletin of the World Health Organization*, 81. © Copyright World Health Organization (WHO). All rights reserved; Figure 3.9: Eye of Science/Science Photo Library; Figure 3.11: Jo Halliday; Figure 3.12: Greg Allgood/Procter and Gamble; Figure 3.14a: Diane Diederich/istockphoto; Figure 3.16: Ronn Altig, University of California, Berkeley; Figure 3.18: WHO/TDR/Martel; Figure 3.19: Bumb, B. and Baanante, C. (1996) *Trends in Fertilizer Use and Projections to 2020*, Brief no. 38, International Food Policy Research Institute; Figure 3.21: Michael Marten/Science Photo Library.

# INDEX

Entries and page numbers in **bold type** refer to key words which are printed in **bold** in the text. Indexed information on pages indicated by *italics* is carried mainly or wholly in a figure or a table.